A Handbook of Clinical Skills

Jane Dacre, BSc MD
FRCP (London, Glasgow)
Professor of Medical Education,
Consultant Physician and Rheumatologist,
Royal Free and University College
Medical School, London, UK

Peter Kopelman, MD FRCP
Professor of Clinical Medicine,
Barts & The London, Queen Mary's
School of Medicine & Dentistry,
University of London, UK

MANSON

To

Nigel, Claire, Robert and Anna
Sue, Sarah, Claire and Tom

For full details of all Manson Publishing Ltd titles please write to:
Manson Publishing Ltd
73 Corringham Road
London NW11 7DL, United Kingdom

Tel: +44(0)20 8905 5150
Fax: +44(0)20 8201 9233

E-mail: manson@man-pub.demon.co.uk
Website: www.manson-publishing.co.uk

Commissioning editor: Jill Northcott
Layout and design: Patrick Daly
Colour reproduction: Acumen Colour Ltd, London, UK
Printed by: Grafos SA, Barcelona, Spain

Contents

Preface

The three most important skills required for day-to-day medical practice are obtaining a comprehensive history, examining a patient correctly and performing simple practical procedures. Mastery of these skills enables a clinician to bring a reasoned approach to the possible diagnosis and management of a patient. They are also a source of continuing enjoyment and challenge.

Although it is sometimes easier to request a long list of investigations, the good clinician is often able to resolve complicated clinical problems quickly and simply, based on a thorough clinical history and examination, followed by a smaller list of *appropriate* investigations. In short, competence in clinical method is a major contributor to excellence in practice.

Our objective in this book is to provide a brief, readable introduction to these important skills: how they can be mastered and how they may then be applied. We have been careful to emphasize communication skills and a respectful approach towards the patient. The book is aimed at all young clinicians who are likely to perform these skills in training, for examination purposes and in practice.

The book begins with an overview of the general examination, followed by chapters on each of the body systems in turn. It includes chapters on the female and male reproductive systems, child health and psychiatry, to apply the principles of clinical method across many disciplines. Although the emphasis is on normal examination, each chapter includes a section on the care of patients with problems related to that particular body system. The book also includes photographs and other illustrations of common medical conditions, and is intentionally pocket sized, so that it can easily be used for reference in the clinical setting.

The book is intended as a practical manual of clinical method, designed to assist the learning clinician within the environment of a hospital or general practice.

It is our sincere hope that use of the book will instil a fascination for clinical practice that remains evident in all of the contributing authors, many years after graduation.

Jane Dacre
Peter Kopelman

Contributors

Philip L. Beales, BSc MD MRCP
Clinical Lecturer in Molecular Medicine and Honorary Consultant in Clinical Genetics, Institute of Child Health and Guy's Hospital, London, UK.

Stephen Brearley, MB MA MChir FRCS
Consultant Vascular Surgeon, Department of Surgery and Urology, Whipps Cross University Hospital, UK.

Jane Dacre, BSc MD FRCP (London, Glasgow)
Professor of Medical Education, Consultant Physician and Rheumatologist, Royal Free and University College Medical School, London, UK.

Peter Kopelman, MD FRCP
Professor of Clinical Medicine, Deputy Warden, Barts & The London, Queen Mary's School of Medicine and Dentistry, London, UK.

Clive Spence-Jones, FRCS MRCOG
Consultant Gynaecologist, Whittington Hospital, London, UK.

Mark Weaver, MBBS MRCPsych
Senior Registrar in Psychiatry, Department of Pyschological Medicine, St. Bartholomew's Hospital Medical College, London, UK.

Peter D. White, BSc MD FRCP FRCPsych
Senior Lecturer in Psychological Medicine, St Bartholomew's Hospital Medical College, London, UK.

Jennifer G. Worrall MD FRCP
Consultant Physician and Rheumatologist, Whittington Hospital, London, UK.

1 History taking and examination

The outcome of a consultation is different for doctor and patient, because each has different objectives. The patient may have come simply to be given a diagnosis, or may be in need of reassurance that all is well physically, or may have a more complicated psychosocial problem that needs to be assessed. The doctor's objective is to explore the patient's problems, decide whether there is a hidden agenda or not, make a diagnostic hypothesis, and offer advice on the next steps that need to be taken.

If the doctor recognizes the pattern of the patient's illness, the diagnosis may be quick and simple. If not, there is a need to expand the history with repeated checking, confirmation and rejection of diagnostic hypotheses. In the majority of cases, the patient's problem becomes apparent during this process.

All patients must be examined: in some cases the diagnosis is only made after physical examination with the interpretation of clinical signs, and/or with diagnostic test results and interpretation of investigations. During the examination procedure, the doctor is considering and confirming or refuting the diagnostic hypothesis that he/she has made.

The three sources of information that are helpful for evaluating a patient's problems and for making a diagnostic hypothesis are:

- The history – this is the patient's account of their illness or presenting complaint, including their reasons for visiting their doctor.
- The clinical signs – these include the abnormalities found on examination.
- The results of initial investigations which may include biochemical and haematological and imaging results.

Throughout this book we will draw attention to these three important areas. In most patients, the process of problem-solving will involve the sequence of history → signs → investigation, but this may not always be so. In some patients it is immediately obvious that it will either be extremely difficult, or even impossible, to obtain a history (e.g. following a cerebrovascular accident). In such circumstances it is appropriate to proceed to the examination, although it is always important to try to obtain a history from someone, a relative, witness or even the ambulance driver.

There are some procedures which must be carried out routinely when examining every patient, while there are others which are used only when there is a special indication – these will be highlighted in the chapters of this book. In taking the history, there are a number of routine questions that must be asked of every patient, e.g. those which concern past illnesses, while the questions relating to the present illness will vary according to the problem. Similarly, certain examination procedures should always be carried out during the clinical examination – for example, measuring the blood pressure, while others are carried out only when certain abnormalities are anticipated – for example, a vaginal examination. You will need to be able to identify the clues which may be provided from the history and the examination. You will need to keep your wits about you as you progress through your assessment, making diagnostic hypotheses, and refuting them. This will enable areas to be identified which may require closer analysis during the examination. You will learn best by witnessing as much as possible in the clinical setting and thereby learning from experience. Do not cut corners as you are learning to apply the techniques of clinical examination.

The practice of history taking (1) and examination varies between clinicians, and so you may see a number of slightly different techniques applied. It is a good idea to discuss any variability that you see, and decide on an appropriate method to fit in with your practice.

Finally, much of the basis of clinical medicine has evolved over several hundred years, so there is a wealth of experience, but little evidence base for clinical method at the present time.

Remember – medicine is an art as well as a science: you may see experts take short cuts in their assessment of patients. This is because experienced clinicians often work using pattern recognition – but you need to have enormous experience before you can do this reliably.

History taking

There should be several different processes going on in your mind while taking a history. The most obvious of these is to form a diagnostic hypothesis as outlined, or an impression about the patient and his/her problems.

History taking skills

- Communication.
- Data gathering, assimilation, and processing.
- Following an accepted structure.
- Forming a diagnosis and developing a plan of action.
- Writing it down.
- Presenting the history to others.

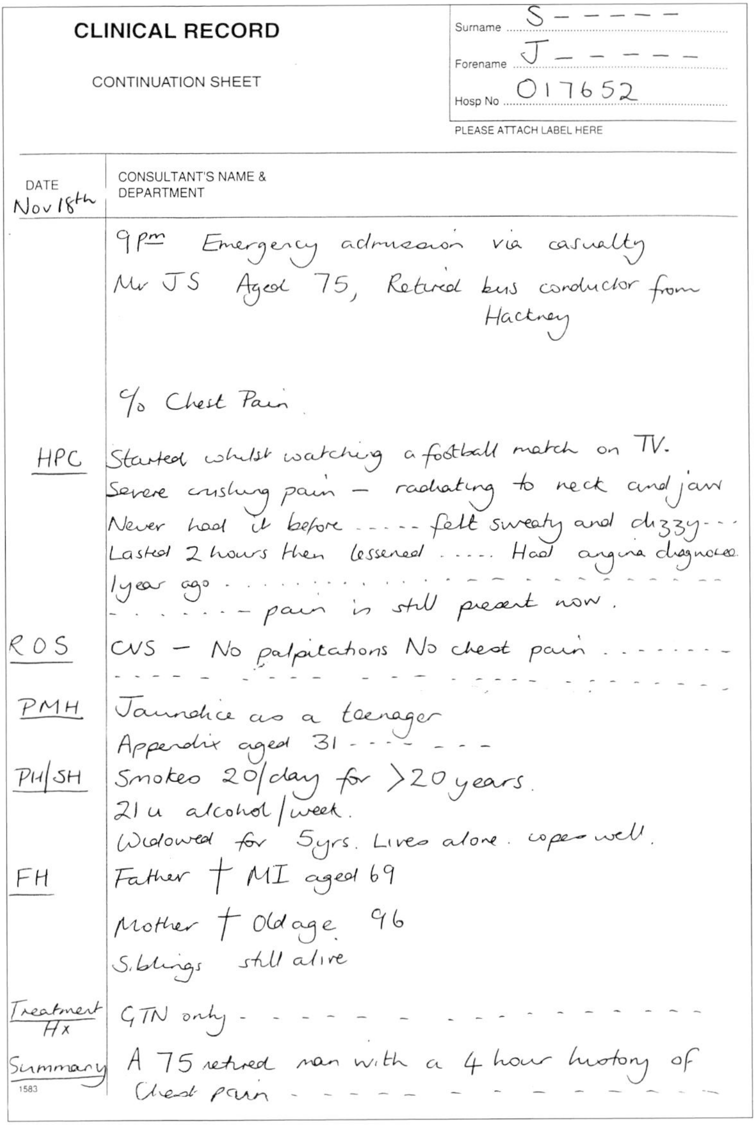

CLINICAL RECORD	Surname ...... S _ _ _ _ _
CONTINUATION SHEET	Forename ...... J _ _ _ _ _
	Hosp No O17652
	PLEASE ATTACH LABEL HERE

DATE Nov 18th	CONSULTANT'S NAME & DEPARTMENT

9 pm   Emergency admission via casualty
Mr JS Aged 75, Retired bus conductor from
                                                  Hackney

C/o Chest Pain

HPC Started whilst watching a football match on TV.
Severe crushing pain — radiating to neck and jaw
Never had it before ..... felt sweaty and dizzy ...
Lasted 2 hours then lessened ..... Had angina diagnosed
1 year ago .... ─ ─ ─ ─
.... ─ pain is still present now.

ROS CVS — No palpitations No chest pain ....
─ ─ ─ ─ ─ ─ ─ ─ ─ ─ ─ ─ ─ ─ ─ ─

PMH Jaundice as a teenager
Appendix aged 31 .... ─ ─ ─

PH/SH Smokes 20/day for >20 years.
21 u alcohol/week.
Widowed for 5yrs. Lives alone. copes well.

FH Father † MI aged 69

Mother † Old age. 96
Siblings still alive

Treatment Hx GTN only ─ ─ ─ ─ ─ ─ ─ ─ ─ ─ ─ ─ ─ ─ ─

Summary A 75 retired man with a 4 hour history of
1583 Chest pain ─ ─ ─ ─ ─ ─ ─ ─ ─ ─ ─

1 Handwritten history of a patient with chest pain.

Communication

The consultation is a time when you develop your relationship with the patient. You need to establish rapport and gain trust. You must make the patient feel comfortable talking about him/herself. Good communication, with careful formulation of questions and reflection of emotions, facilitates the patient in telling you all the information you need. The quality of your explanations helps the patient to trust your advice and decision making.

General advice

Always try to be polite – never talk to a patient without first introducing yourself, and then asking permission to perform an examination. Explain why you want to talk to him/her. Often, students are embarrassed talking to patients because they feel they have nothing to offer. However, if the patient is told the purpose of the encounter, they very rarely object and often welcome the interest.

Be aware that most patients expect an appropriate appearance from a professional person. Make sure that you dress in a way which you believe a patient will expect of a doctor, i.e. neat, clean, and conventional. Very fashionable clothing is often inappropriate. Always address the patient as Mr, Mrs or Miss unless asked to do otherwise. Avoid terms like 'dear'. Do not continue if the patient is tired – and do not embark on lengthy history taking sessions at mealtimes or when the patient has visitors. Find times when the patients are free and come back. You will get a better history if they are not preoccupied.

The interviewer should guide the patient over the relevant areas of enquiry, striking a balance between the need to collect information in the time available and the wish to carry out the interview in a manner the patient finds most comfortable.

Be aware of non-verbal signals and body language. Good eye contact (i.e. looking at the patient as you speak to him/her), an appropriate space between you, and mirroring the patient's posture can encourage the patient to speak more freely and help develop trust. Adopt an 'open' posture (2) so the patient is encouraged to talk to you. Make it obvious that you are listening (3) by perhaps occasionally leaning forward and putting your hand on your chin. Make sure that you are sitting at the same level as the patient: it is intimidating for the patient to be lying in bed with the doctor standing over them. Make sure that you are at an appropriate distance – about an arm's length away. Make use of touch – you must find a level at which you feel comfortable touching the patient – decide whether you are the kind of person who wants to shake the patient's hand, or put your hand on his/her shoulder (4). If you or the patient finds this uncomfortable, touch the hand or elbow as this is less intimidating. Make eye contact regularly – do not just look down at your notes – and interact with the patient by smiling, or showing sympathy if sad things are discussed.

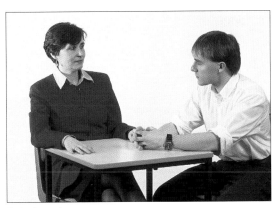

2 An 'open' posture.

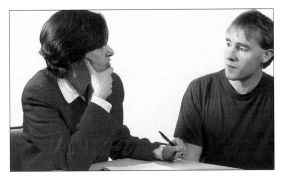

3 A 'listening' posture.

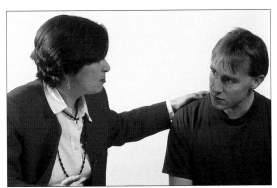

4 Appropriate use of touch.

Spoken communication

Always ensure that you speak clearly, and avoid the use of jargon. Do not use technical or ambiguous wording. Encourage the patients to talk about his/her problems. It's best to ask as many open questions as possible, especially at the start of the interview, to enable the patient to tell you what is wrong in his/her own words. This enhances trust and confidence, as the patient will feel you are listening and therefore taking him/her seriously. Closed questions are needed to direct the interview and to explore abnormal experiences. Always try to open the question again to clarify the response, for example:

'Have you had the feeling, perhaps, that it is brought on by anything in particular?' (closed)

'Could you tell me something about that?' (open)

Leading questioning, in which there is an expectation of a particular response, should only be used to clarify an uncertain answer, e.g.: 'Your appetite's been poor, hasn't it?', or 'You've lost weight, haven't you?'

It is usually helpful to begin the consultation with an open question (**Table 1**), such as 'What exactly brought you into hospital?' You should ensure that the patient replies by describing the presenting symptoms or worries and *not* the eventual diagnosis, e.g. angina or bronchitis.

It is useful in this context to use words such as 'How?' and 'Why'. For example, 'How can I help you?', 'How does if affect you?'. In this way, it is difficult for the patient to give a one-word answer, and they have to describe the problem. If you use phrases such as: 'Do you have a pain in your chest?', the patient may just say 'Yes' – and tell you nothing more.

Try not to interrupt at the beginning of the history. Use techniques like nodding and saying 'I see', or paraphrase the patient's last statement. Once you have the patient talking, you must listen to what they say and follow his/her story, and explore the problem. Only then can you begin to concentrate on your own agenda, and ask more direct, or focused questions, either leading or closed. Begin by reiterating the patients' phrases and checking your understanding of them: 'You say the pain felt like a band – what sort of band?'. Then move to direct questions to elicit more specific information – 'Did the pain go anywhere else?', 'Where?', 'Did it make you sweat?'. Try to show respect, and be non-judgmental towards whatever the patient is telling you. Be careful not to stop listening.

Table 1. Useful phrases in open questioning

- 'How can I help you?'
- 'What can I do for you?'
- 'Why did you …?'
- 'Tell me about …'
- 'Can you describe it?'
- 'Where did …?'
- 'What is it like?'
- 'When did …?'

Empathic statements

These can convey an acknowledgement of the patient's problems and may enable an inhibited patient to expand on a topic which is difficult for him or her to discuss openly.

- 'I can understand that this may be difficult for you but ...'(before asking a question).
- 'I can see that this is causing you distress.'
- 'I can see you've been under a lot of stress.'

Clarification

- 'I'm not entirely clear what you mean by ...'
- 'Could you tell me a little more about ...'

Remarks on behaviour

Made during the interview, these can help explore important areas, or perhaps defuse a difficult situation.

- 'You seemed quite sad/angry/distressed when you talked about ...'

Enabling statements

- 'It is not uncommon when under a lot of stress to experience intense or strange feelings or worries. Has anything like this been happening to you?' The patient may then be asked to elaborate.

Controlling

This can be done during natural silences or by gently interrupting at an appropriate point.

- 'I hate to interrupt, but can you tell me more about ...'
- 'I'd like to move on, if I may ...'
- 'I'm sorry, but I need to know more about this' (change topic).

Silences

A brief and well-timed period of silence can allow a patient space to elaborate about a painful topic. Allow a patient time to gather his/her thoughts – and don't be afraid to interrupt and redirect him or her if he/she are getting away from the subject – but beware of allowing long, embarrassing silences. Once you feel confident with using this style and pattern of question it is possible to concentrate on the next stage of history taking and data gathering.

Data gathering and assimilation

It is important to keep your eyes open, as well as to listen attentively, when taking the history – and to remember that you are gathering information throughout the encounter. Physical signs may be observed while taking the history, or an unexpected finding during the later examination may require you to return to the history and re-analyse a particular area. The diagnostic value of the history will vary from patient to patient, and is generally dependent upon the patient's presenting complaint. A complaint of chest pain should trigger a series of questions related to the possible causes, whereas a complaint of tiredness may be less clear-cut. Some patients are naturally good historians, while others will find it difficult to describe the problems.

Be aware that some patients will inadvertently select information which he/she think you should know and thereby present a somewhat false picture of the complaints. Similarly, you may not pick up the clues provided by other patients and fail to ask the right questions. It is helpful to summarize your understanding of what you have been told – and relay it back to the patient:

'I understand the pain lasted about two hours, is that right?'

This checks for accuracy and completeness. It is always important when you are first taking a history to be prepared to go back to the patient after you have finished the history if you realize that you have omitted a vital point. Don't jump to conclusions during the history taking, and avoid rationalizing the different parts in order to fit a specific diagnosis you have in mind. You must explore every possibility – even an apparently straightforward history may have a twist. This underlines the value of problem listing at the end of the history taking and examination.

Following an accepted structure

The ability to take an efficient and accurate history will come only with experience. Table 2 provides general guidance to enable you to cover the important areas and collect the relevant data: you are advised to follow the order of the topics whenever you write out a history, although the information may not come from the patient in that order.

There will be occasions when it is not appropriate to take a comprehensive history at the time you first see the patient. The patient in cardiogenic shock will need immediate treatment, as will the patient with a perforated peptic ulcer. A good general knowledge of medicine is required to enable you to judge when it is important to take a detailed history and when it is sufficient to question simply about the immediate presenting complaint.

You may see senior colleagues cutting corners – but it is not advisable to do this yourself until you are experienced enough to know what to leave out. They are using their clinical experience to do this – it is not wise to follow that example until you have a similar degree of expertise.

Table 2. Following an accepted structure

- Name, age, etc.
- Presenting complaint
- The history of the present illness
- Past medical history
- Systems review
- Personal and social history
- Family history and treatment history

Table 3. Ways of encouraging the patient's description of their presenting complaint	
Location	Point to it?
Radiation	Does it spread anywhere?
Duration	How long has it been present? Have you had anything like this before?
Timing	Is it there all the time or does it come and go? If it comes and goes, how long do you get it?
Nature	What sort of pain is it? Is it burning, stabbing, gripping, etc.?
Severity	How bad is it? Does it stop you working or keep you awake at night?
Precipitating/ alleviating factors	Is there anything which makes it better or worse?
Associated symptoms	Do you have any other associated symptoms?

History of presenting complaint

Begin by listening to the patient's own account, asking questions around particular areas. This account may already suggest to you possible causes for the patient's problem and likely reactions to your information or advice. Your intent with supplementary questions should be to analyse such possibilities and deal with the reactions.

Once the patient has described the presenting problem(s), you should try to establish more precisely the exact nature, severity, and timing of the symptoms.

You must enquire whether the patient has ever experienced similar symptoms in the past. If so, you must explore the relevant history.

Continuously analyse the patient's symptoms (see **Table 3**) and answers to your questions, considering the various conditions which might account for them. This will lead you to ask additional specific questions – guidance about such questions will be provided in the history sections of the succeeding chapters.

Table 4. Systems review topics

Remember to ask these questions in language the patient can understand

General	Body weight – has there been a recent change? Appetite, fever?
Respiratory system	Cough and sputum; haemoptysis; dyspnoea; chest pain?
Cardiovascular system	Dyspnoea on exertion; nocturnal dyspnoea; chest pain; ankle swelling; palpitations?
Gastrointestinal	Indigestion; abdominal pain; nausea or vomiting; constipation or diarrhoea; passing blood in the motions?
Urinary	Frequency of micturition; pain on urination (dysuria); passing blood in the urine; nocturia; difficulty in passing urine?
Nervous system	Headaches; disturbance of consciousness (faints or fits); disturbance of vision or hearing; disturbance of limb function?
Locomotion	Pain or stiffness in muscles or joints?
Menstrual function	Usual rhythm (duration of each period and length of cycle); disturbance of rhythm; excessive blood loss; post-menopausal bleeding?
Allergies	Urticaria; hay-fever; specific allergies, in particular to drugs?
Drugs	Any drugs or medicines currently being taken or taken in the recent past, including 'over-the-counter' medications; abnormal reactions to drugs, e.g. reactions to antibiotics?

Systems review

The next step is to ask questions about the presence or absence of symptoms relating to all systems (review of systems) which have not been touched upon in the first part of the history. This routine enquiry is designed not only to reveal additional symptoms or problems related to the presenting illness, but also to uncover symptoms resulting from other unsuspected disorders. The check list will usually include questions covering the points shown in **Table 4**. Some clinicians prefer to ask these questions at the end of the history – the timing is a matter of personal preference.

Past medical history

Some aspects of the past medical history may have already been obtained. Nevertheless, try to obtain more detailed information about any serious illness or surgical operations in the past. It is helpful to record the dates of the illness/operation and the hospitals which the patient attended. It is also useful to check whether the patient has had any medical examinations in the past for insurance reasons, and the outcome of the assessment. Finally, trips abroad and details of immunizations are sometimes relevant, particularly in the case of a suspected infectious disease.

Personal and social history

Ask about the patient's social circumstances – marital status, what is his/her occupation, and where does he/she live? An enquiry about the home in relation to heating, sanitation, and other facilities may be relevant. Always ask patients about smoking and drinking habits. Alcohol intake should be recorded as units per week; a unit is 1 measure of spirit, a glass of wine or 0.25 L of beer. It is also helpful to enquire about eating habits, particularly if you suspect a nutritional deficiency. It may sometimes be appropriate to enquire if the patient uses recreational drugs.

The social history often offers the interviewer an opportunity to get to know the patient better, but can obviously be a sensitive area of enquiry. It is important that you are aware of such sensitivities and use common sense when asking questions. However, do not be reluctant to enquire about the patient's current or past occupations – it is sometimes fascinating to learn of a patient's background and their skills. A suggested general line of questioning is shown on the opposite page. You may begin, for example, with the patient's occupation.

Try to ensure that you use your communication skills to explore areas of concern, and follow the leads that the patient offers you.

While you are taking the history, you may become aware that the patient is very anxious or unduly depressed by his/her situation. It is appropriate to ask the patient whether they are worried about anything or depressed – refer to Chapter 11 for guidance about taking a psychiatric history.

Personal and social history: questions to ask

● 'What is your occupation … describe your job to me … what do you do during a normal day … can you manage it without any difficulty?'

Then enquire about the patient's home life, to assess whether the illness has affected his/her ability to cope at home:

● 'Where do you live … in a house or flat … do you own it … are you up to date with the rent … how many stairs are there … can you get up and down them OK … can you cope with the housework … do you have any help … who is it from … do you have any social service support … who is at home with you … is he/she fit … does he/she help you … are any relatives near you … do they help you out … do you have local friends?'

Family and treatment history

You should enquire about the health of parents and siblings: 'Are your parents still alive?' … 'What did they die from?' and whether there is any family history of particular illnesses. It is important to note whether there is a family history of death at an early age from heart disease. You should also detail the recent and past treatment history, allergies to or adverse effects from particular treatments, and whether the patient has taken any 'over-the-counter' preparations – try to record the generic rather than proprietary ('drug company') names of drugs where possible. This is a useful habit for later.

When you have completed taking the history, you should have elicited some clues to the main causes of the patient's problems. The history may have indicated the system(s) which will require particular attention during the examination. If no such clues have come to light, then a more detailed general examination is essential.

The routine physical examination

The details of the various examinations you should perform are described in the chapters of this book. This section will summarize a system for performing a routine physical examination. While you are learning the system for clinical examination it is important to perform a complete examination as often as possible. This will ensure that the scheme becomes second nature to you and should prevent you making serious omissions. You are strongly advised to return to your patient if you find that you have omitted a part of the examination – most patients will not mind this, providing that you are honest. This will ensure that you remember that area of the examination next time. In the routine examination of each system only certain assessments are performed as a routine unless an abnormality is found. If anything abnormal is found, then additional tests or analysis is needed: an example is the series of manoeuvres required if a heart murmur is heard (see Chapter 2). You will find that the time you take to perform the general examination will be within acceptable limits once you have perfected the technique.

Scheme for the routine physical examination

Ensure that you maintain the patient's privacy as much as possible throughout the examination, and do not do anything without asking the patient first. Always be polite and considerate. Give clear instructions about what you want the patient to do – they are unlikely to be familiar with some of the actions which you request. Although it is possible to perform a full examination by considering each system in turn, this is not recommended as it causes unnecessary duplication. It is more logical to start by observing the patient's general appearance and then to examine the hands, the face and head, neck, chest, abdomen, joints, and finally the nervous system. Within the systems, follow the scheme: inspection, palpation, percussion, auscultation.

General observation

You should observe the patient's gait and ability to perform coordinated movements. While taking the history, you should note the patient's mental alertness and intelligence. You should also observe the patient's body build, muscularity and the condition of the skin (rashes, pigmentation, etc.). If the patient feels febrile, or gives a history of fever, then the oral temperature should be taken.

Table 5. Checklist for the routine physical examination

- General observations (inspection)
- Hands and arms
- Head and neck, including lymph nodes, breasts and thyroid
- Heart and chest
- Abdomen
- Legs, including joints
- Nervous system

Hands and arms

Look for finger clubbing and examine the nails – excessive brittleness may reflect iron deficiency, whereas white nails (leukonychia) is a sign of chronic liver disease. Look at the skin creases in the palms of the hands for evidence of anaemia or pigmentation and any other abnormalities. Note any wasting of the muscles of the hands or arms, and look for swelling of the joints and limitation of movement. Feel the radial pulse and note the rhythm and rate. Measure the blood pressure; palpate the axillae and epitrochlear regions for enlarged lymph glands and note the presence or absence of axillary hair. Ask the patient to hold his/her arms out in front and check for a tremor of the outstretched fingers.

Head and neck

Look at the sclerae of the eyes for jaundice, and the conjunctiva for anaemia. Examine the teeth, the tongue and the mouth and look at the fauces, noting the presence or absence of the tonsils. Look at the buccal mucosa for evidence of hyperpigmentation. Examine the neck for cervical and supraclavicular lymphadenopathy and determine whether the thyroid is palpable. You should examine the breasts in women for any swellings, masses or tenderness.

Chest and heart

Estimate the central venous pressure by inspection of the internal jugular vein. Locate the carotid arteries and note their character and whether they are equal in pulsation. Feel for the apex beat, and then palpate and assess whether the left or right ventricle is enlarged. Listen to the heart sounds and the presence of any murmurs – use the flat of your hand to detect any palpable thrills.

Observe the chest movement and use your hands to confirm its symmetry. Palpate the trachea and locate its position. Percuss over the lungs on the front and sides of the chest and then auscultate over the front of the chest. Now sit the patient forward looking for any deformities of the chest or spine. Percuss and listen over the back of the chest; concentrate particularly at the lung bases for any added sounds such as crackles, and listen for vocal fremitus. While the patient is leaning forward you must examine the sacral region for any evidence of oedema.

Abdomen

Observe the general appearance of the abdomen, looking for distension, peristalsis, dilated veins, and any obvious enlargement of viscera or abnormal masses. Palpate the abdomen gently and then more deeply, feeling for the spleen, the liver, and left and right kidneys. Look for enlargement of the inguinal glands and feel the femoral pulses. Examine the hernial orifices and the external genitalia in men. Listen to the bowel sounds and listen over the aorta and renal arteries. Consider a rectal examination.

Legs

You should examine the legs, looking for abnormalities such as wasting, swelling of the ankles, varicose veins, and tenderness in the calves. You should also examine the joints for swelling or limitation of movement. You should note the state of the circulation, feeling whether the limbs are warm or unduly cold – feel for the popliteal, posterior tibial, and dorsalis pedis arterial pulses.

Nervous system

You will have noted already the patient's appearance and intelligence – if you suspect confusion or an impairment of mental function, then more detailed questioning will be appropriate (see Chapter 6). Ask the patient whether he/she is right- or left-handed. Test the cranial nerves and look at the fundi and eardrums. Test motor function in the upper and lower limbs, including the tendon and plantar reflex responses, and follow this by assessing sensation (pinprick and vibration sense). Finally, assess the patient's ability to perform coordinated movements. Ideally, you should examine the nervous system in detail when you are learning because it is a useful way of gaining experience of the wide range of normality for the many signs elicited.

An example of examination findings written in the patient's notes is shown in 5–7.

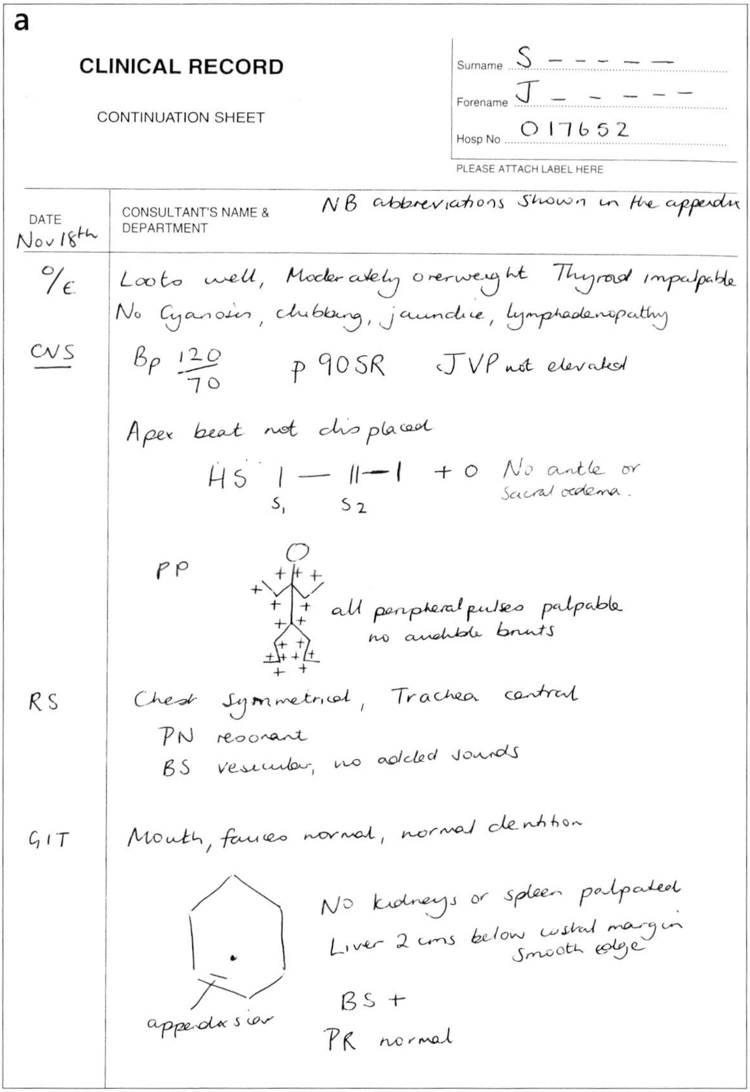

a

CLINICAL RECORD

CONTINUATION SHEET

Surname ...S. _ _ _ _ _

Forename ...J _ _ _ _ _ _

Hosp No ...O 1 7 6 5 2

PLEASE ATTACH LABEL HERE

DATE Nov 18th	CONSULTANT'S NAME & DEPARTMENT	NB abbreviations shown in the appendix

O/E — Looks well, Moderately overweight   Thyroid impalpable
No Cyanosis, clubbing, jaundice, lymphadenopathy

CVS — Bp $\frac{120}{70}$ p 90 SR   JVP not elevated

Apex beat not displaced

HS 1 — II — 1   + O   No ankle or
      S₁   S₂   Sacral oedema.

PP   all peripheral pulses palpable
         no audible bruits

RS — Chest symmetrical, Trachea central
PN resonant
BS vesicular, no added sounds

GIT — Mouth, fauces normal, normal dentition

      No kidneys or spleen palpated
      Liver 2 cms below costal margin
                           Smooth edge

appendix scar   BS +
                   PR normal

5 Examination findings as written in clinical notes – CVS, Rs, GIT.

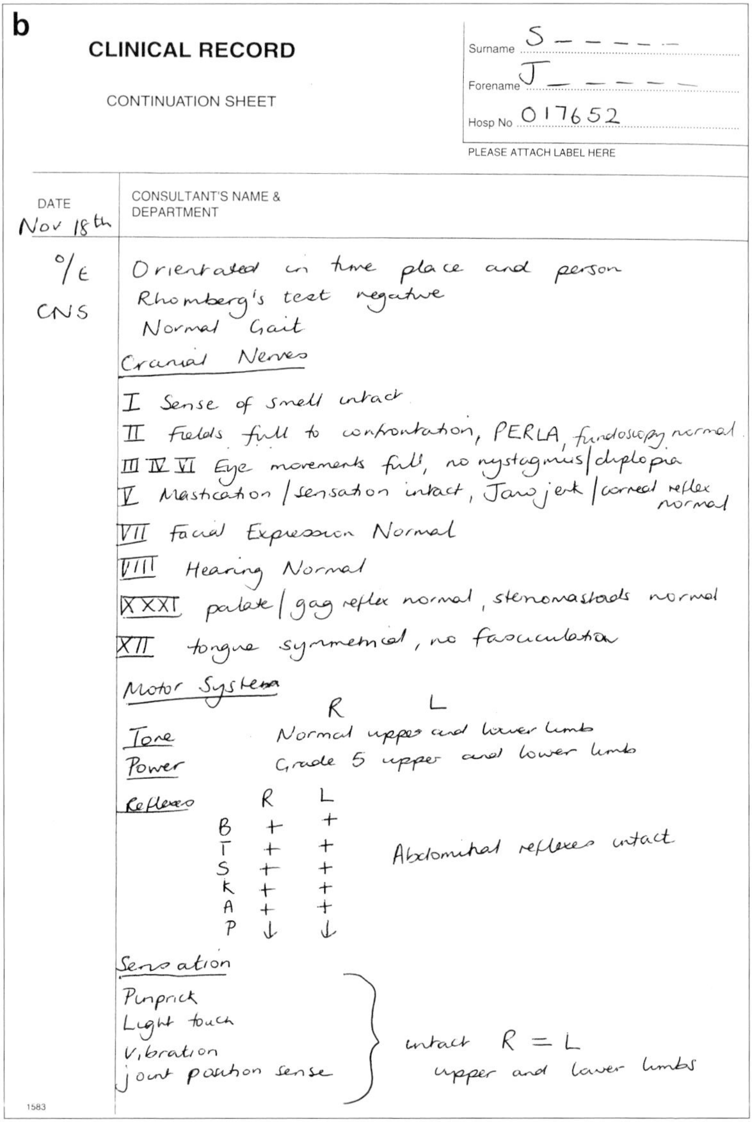

b

CLINICAL RECORD

CONTINUATION SHEET

Surname S _ _ _ _ _

Forename J _ _ _ _ _

Hosp No 017652

PLEASE ATTACH LABEL HERE

DATE
Nov 18th

CONSULTANT'S NAME & DEPARTMENT

O/E

CNS

Orientated in time place and person
Rhomberg's test negative
Normal Gait

Cranial Nerves

I   Sense of smell intact.

II Fields full to confrontation, PERLA, fundoscopy normal.

III IV VI Eye movements full, no nystagmus/diplopia

V   Mastication/sensation intact, Jaw jerk/corneal reflex
    normal

VII Facial Expression Normal

VIII Hearing Normal

IX X XI palate/gag reflex normal, sternomastoids normal

XII tongue symmetrical, no fasciculation

Motor System

		R	L
Tone		Normal upper and lower limbs	
Power		Grade 5 upper and lower limbs	

Reflexes

	R	L	
B	+	+	
T	+	+	Abdominal reflexes intact
S	+	+	
K	+	+	
A	+	+	
P	↓	↓	

Sensation

Pinprick
Light touch
Vibration
joint position sense

intact R = L
upper and lower limbs

1583

6 Examination findings as written in clinical notes – CNS.

C		
CLINICAL RECORD	Surname	S _ _ _ _ _
	Forename	J _ _ _ _ _
CONTINUATION SHEET	Hosp No	017652
	PLEASE ATTACH LABEL HERE	

DATE	CONSULTANT'S NAME & DEPARTMENT

Co - ordination

Finger / nose test normal

Heel / shin test normal

Locomotor System

	R	L	
G	✓	✓	
A	✓	✓	Normal appearance and movement
L	✓	✓	
S	✓	✓	

Summary 75 year old man with ischaemic
Sounding chest pain. Risk factors: Smoking
Normal examination
Impression

MI
Unstable Angina

Plan   ECG   Cardiac Enzymes
          CXR
          FBC   Signed: JMJ.
                             Date: Nov 18ᵀᴴ

7 Examination findings as written in clinical notes – locomotor system diagram.

Formulating a diagnosis

Towards the completion of your history, you must ask yourself what the diagnosis is. Make a diagnostic hypothesis – and then confirm or refute this by asking further questions.

In some patients, the diagnosis is obvious. This is called a 'spot diagnosis', and is based on pattern recognition, for example, a child with a fever, a vesicular rash, and a history of a brother with chicken pox. Under these circumstances, the history and examination still need to be taken to help manage the case appropriately.

In a more complex case, a more detailed history is necessary to allow you to formulate a diagnostic hypothesis. For example, in a patient with joint pain, if it affects several small joints, the diagnosis is more likely to be an inflammatory arthritis. If it affects a small number of large joints it is likely to be degenerative. If the joints are stiff in the mornings, there is a *possibility* of inflammatory arthritis; if they are stiff in the evenings, the cause is *more likely* to be degenerative ... and so on. The diagnosis is made by matching the history from your patient with your knowledge of the pattern of the condition in your current diagnostic hypothesis. Eventually you come up with what you believe to be the most likely diagnosis. A scheme for this kind of thinking is shown in **8**.

Writing it down

At the same time as taking the history it is important to record the findings in an ordered way. Do not forget to put the date and time of the interview – this is a vital point of history recording which has considerable medico-legal importance. In addition, make sure the name of the patient is recorded at the top of every page. An example of this is shown in **1**. This enables you to use your notes to present the patient to your colleagues, and acts as a prompt and aide memoire to you – and a lead to others treating the same patient.

It is acceptable to use some abbreviations in your note-keeping. A list of those more commonly used is in the Glossary on pages 311–313.

Finally, remember that you should be considering and refuting diagnostic hypotheses throughout the history-taking process – it is worthwhile recording some of this process as an 'impression' or 'summary' section in the notes before recording the physical findings. This helps you and your colleagues to understand your line of thought.

Remember always to sign and date all your entries at the end. Make sure that your writing is legible, and that your status is documented.

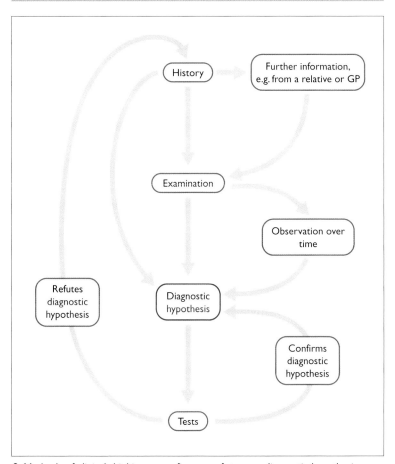

8 Methods of clinical thinking to confirm or refute your diagnostic hypothesis.

Presenting your findings to others

Presenting findings to colleagues This is an important part of patient care, and is often assessed in medical student and postgraduate examinations.

You should speak clearly – and have a clear summary of the patient's problems in your head. Remember that body language and eye contact are as important in presenting your findings as they are in taking the history. People often have a problem with what to do with their hands while presenting a history. It is good advice to decide where you will put them beforehand – and perhaps use them to illustrate a point – or gesture towards the patient – or even hold your notes!

You must be able to re-order the information given to you in the structure outlined above, and summarize the most important points, mentioning any relevant negative findings and all of your positive findings. Then present and discuss your diagnostic hypothesis. For example, from the history written down for 1 (page 9), you might make a verbal presentation along the following lines:

Verbal presentation

'Mr J.S. is a 75-year-old retired bus conductor who presented with his first episode of severe chest pain. It lasted for 2 hours and made him feel sweaty. It radiated to his neck and jaw. A diagnosis of angina was made a year ago. The pain was still there when he arrived.'

- *Then continue with a summary of the relevant risk factors:*

'He is a smoker of 20 cigarettes per day, and has a family history of ischaemic heart disease. We do not know his cholesterol level, and he is not hypertensive.'

- *Continue with the findings:*

'On examination, he looked well. His blood pressure was 120/80 mmHg. General examination was normal. In his cardiovascular system, his pulse was 80 in sinus rhythm, he was not in heart failure…'

- *Then mention your diagnostic hypothesis:*

'I think he has acute coronary syndrome.'

Problem-oriented medical records

Some clinicians prefer to present their findings in a problem oriented way.

The purpose of problem-oriented medical records (POMR) is to structure the medical case history to make it easier to interpret the relevant clinical information, and to provide a framework for planning diagnostic tests and therapeutic procedures. It will also help to remind you – the clinician – what is troubling your patient and how such problems may be resolved.

The emphasis of POMR is the compilation of a list of problems on the basis of the clinical findings (history and examination). The diagnosis or diagnoses, will only be made if *all* problems are considered. If used appropriately, POMR will help you to make decisions about patient care; it will also provide a structure which is very helpful for medical audit.

How to make a problem-oriented medical record

Problem listing: Review your patient's history and examination findings and list all the apparent problems (including social/domestic ones). You should list the problems in what you consider to be an order of priority with the presenting medical problem(s) at the top – P1, P2, P3, etc. Problems may be categorized into 'active' or current problems and 'inactive' or past problems – to recognize possible associations between past and current problems. For example, rheumatic fever as a child may be the explanation for the development of cardiac failure as an adult.

In this circumstance, the presenting problem of breathlessness (P1) should be listed as follows: P1 Breathlessness – past history of rheumatic heart disease. All the problems should be listed, irrespective of whether they are currently active or inactive, if you consider that they may have a bearing on the patient's well-being. For example, if your patient with breathlessness and a past history of rheumatic heart disease has also been treated for a peptic ulcer, this should be listed as a problem, i.e. P2.

This is significant if the patient needs anticoagulation therapy for mitral valve disease – endoscopy should be performed before starting warfarin to confirm the inactivity of the ulcer.

Structuring each problem: Having listed the problems, you should start to formulate an initial plan of investigations and possible treatment. This requires you to think about a possible diagnosis or diagnoses which best fit the clinical findings. It is useful at this stage to analyse each of the patient's main problems in more detail by using the principle of SOAPI. This stands for Subjective, Objective, Assessment, Plan, and (patient) Information – in other words, all the factors you will be considering to make a diagnosis. The box on this page shows the effect of applying SOAPI to our patient with breathlessness.

Progress notes: It is useful to follow the patient's progress during the admission by keeping progress notes in a similar structured fashion, addressing each of the patient's active problems in turn. These should be clearly written, signed, and dated.

P1 Breathlessness – past history of rheumatic fever

S Breathlessness.
O History and clinical signs suggest cardiac failure, raised jugular venous pressure (JVP), bilateral ankle oedema, and basal crepitations. In addition, there is a pansystolic murmur at the apex and atrial fibrillation.
A Biventricular failure possibly secondary to rheumatic valvular disease.
P ECG, chest X-ray (if not already done), blood cultures, and an echocardiogram.
I 'Your breathlessness results from congestion on the lungs due to some heart failure.'

P2 Past history of peptic ulcer disease

S No complaints.
O No symptoms or signs.
A Probably now resolved.
P Needs an endoscopy in view of likely anticoagulation.
I Informed about endoscopic procedure.

General therapeutic and technical skills

The practical skills presented here are those which are commonly used, but do not relate to any one system.

Before discussing specific skills, it is worthwhile thinking about the issue of informed consent (see box below). No procedure may be attempted on a patient unless he/she agrees to have it carried out. With a conscious adult patient who is able to think rationally, the procedure must be discussed before it is attempted. Before larger procedures such as endoscopy or surgery, the patient is required to sign a form documenting their consent. With smaller procedures, verbal consent is adequate.

Only when the patient understands this information is he/she in a position to decide whether or not they wish the procedure to be carried out.

There are several instances of medical litigation relating to patients' lack of understanding of procedures, and their outcome ... so be careful.

Urine testing

At the end of your history and examination you should – if appropriate – test the patient's urine (using a laboratory dipstick) for protein, glucose, and other substances such as urobilinogen. This is a very simple task. Ask the patient to provide you with a mid-stream specimen. Make sure that the dipsticks you use are within date – and follow the instructions on the side of the container.

Informed consent means the patient needs to know:

- The procedure to be undertaken.
- The name of the person who will perform the procedure.
- The likely effects of the procedure (i.e. how will they feel when they wake up; will there be drainage tubes/catheters, etc).
- The possible adverse (but unlikely) effects of the procedure.
- Any likely adverse effects of the procedure.

Phlebotomy: preparing yourself and the patient

- Wash your hands and put on sterile gloves.
- Place the patient's arm in a comfortable position and apply the tourniquet. Make sure you are standing or sitting comfortably, and the patient is either sitting or lying down.
- Look in the antecubital fossa first. Find the vein by feeling over its presumed position. Get a feel for its size, and check its direction.
- Clean the vein with a sterile alcohol swab. Allow the alcohol to dry or wipe with sterile cotton wool. The clean area should be touched as little as possible from now on.

Phlebotomy

Phlebotomy is part of everyday ward life. It is worthwhile practising frequently in order to become really good at it before you qualify. It is a slightly painful procedure for the patient, so they should be warned and asked to keep still during the procedure.

Always introduce yourself and explain what you are going to do, and why. Outline how you will perform the procedure, and ask them if they have any questions. Make sure that you have the patient's verbal consent before you start.

Always check that the patient is not allergic to the drugs/solutions you are going to use. Before beginning any procedure, ensure that all the necessary equipment is there. Check the request form and make sure you have the correct bottles before you start, i.e. syringes, needles, blood bottles, cotton wool, an alcohol swab, and a plaster.

Needles should be carefully disposed of, either by clicking the needle off the syringe by using the keyhole-shaped opening in the top of the sharps bin, and disposing of the syringe in a yellow clinical waste bin, or by disposing of the waste needle and syringe in the sharps container, whichever is appropriate. If this is not possible, i.e. at the bedside, put all your instruments in the cardboard tray and dispose of them as above at the nearest sharps bin. NEVER re-sheath needles. With the needle off the syringe, gently squirt the blood into the correct bottles. Check that you have filled the bottle to the line. Firmly secure the cap, and invert the bottle gently a few times to ensure the blood is mixed with any anticoagulant in the bottle. Finally, ensure that you label the bottle correctly.

Blood sampling using a needle and syringe

- Open the syringe, attach the needle to the syringe by opening the needle cover and pressing it onto the end.
- Push the plunger in as far as it will go to loosen it, and remove all air.
- Secure the skin adjacent to the vessel with your non-dominant thumb.
- Hold the syringe with your index finger pointing towards the needle and enter the skin at an angle of about 45°(**9**). Ensure that the bevel of the needle is pointing upwards. You will feel a pop as you enter the vein.
- Reduce the angle a little and use your non-dominant hand to withdraw the plunger to aspirate the correct amount of blood.
- Remove the tourniquet BEFORE taking the needle out of the vein.
- Apply mild pressure with a cotton wool ball as you withdraw the needle. Ask the patient or your assistant to apply pressure to the site for about 1 minute before applying a plaster.

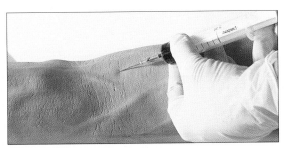

9 Venepuncture.

Blood sampling using a vacutainer system

Many hospitals use a vacutainer system for phlebotomy. With this system, venous access is secured by using a vacutainer needle attached to a plastic, evacuated cylinder. The vacutainer bottles have a rubber bung which is pierced by the distal end of the vacutainer needle.

- The correct amount of blood is drawn into the bottle by the vacuum.
- The bottle is removed when the flow through the needle stops, and the tourniquet released before removing the needle from the arm, as in conventional venepuncture.
- Finally, the vacutainer bottle needs to be inverted to mix its contents with any anticoagulant in the bottle.

Setting up 'the giving set' for intravenous (i.v.) administration

This is a useful skill, seldom taught to doctors. The aim is to set up a bag of fluid attached to an i.v. line containing no bubbles.

- Open the i.v. bag and the giving set, which come in sterile containers.
- Unwind the giving set, and close the adjustable valve.

- Remove the sterile cover from the bag outlet and from the sharp end of the giving set (**10a**). Push the giving set end into the bag outlet. You may need to use quite a lot of force, but be careful not to de-sterilize the end.

- Invert the bag, hang it up on a stand and squeeze the drip chamber to half-fill it with fluid.

- Open the valve partially, to allow the drip to run, and watch the fluid run through to the end. If you do this too quickly, bubbles will collect. They are difficult to get rid of – if they do occur, try tapping or flicking the tubing.

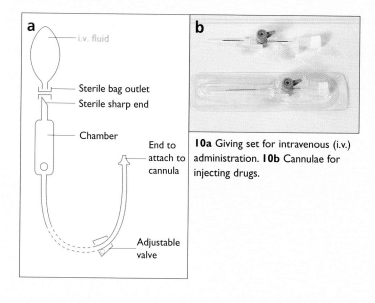

a

i.v. fluid

Sterile bag outlet

Sterile sharp end

Chamber

End to attach to cannula

Adjustable valve

b

10a Giving set for intravenous (i.v.) administration. **10b** Cannulae for injecting drugs.

Preparing an intravenous cannula

Intravenous cannulae are used for patients in whom constant venous access is required. This is because they require frequent intravenous injections, or may need urgent resuscitation. The cannula is left *in situ*, but sealed off with a rubber bung through which access is possible at any time. Before beginning any procedure, ensure you have all the necessary equipment. (This includes local anaesthetic, a supply of three cannulae, an alcohol swab, and tape for fixing the cannula in place.) Carefully remove the cannula from its packaging and check how it works. It consists of a sharp needle surrounded by a plastic sheath. The needle can be withdrawn from the plastic sheath. Some cannulae have side arms for injecting drugs (**10b**).

Always introduce yourself to the patient and explain what you are going to do and why. Outline how you will perform the procedure, and ask if there are any questions. Make sure that you have the patient's verbal consent before you start, and remember to wash your hands and wear sterile disposable gloves.

This can be a painful procedure, so you need the patient's full cooperation if possible. Only attempt cannulation three times at one sitting, as it hurts, and you may lose the patient's cooperation. If you think it will be a difficult cannulation, spend a long time locating the best vein, and use topical local anaesthetic cream applied at least one hour beforehand and, if possible, get expert help.

Procedure for siting an intravenous cannula

● Place the arm in a comfortable position and apply the tourniquet below the elbow. Make sure you are standing or sitting comfortably, and the patient is sitting or lying down.

● Cannulae are best sited in wide straight veins away from joints. There is one of these on the radial side of the wrist. Find the vein by feeling over its presumed position. Get a feel for its size and check the direction in which it is running. Flick or tap it to make it stand out.

● Clean the skin over the area you intend to puncture with a sterile alcohol swab (steret). Allow the alcohol to dry. The clean area should be touched as little as possible from now on. If you are going to inject local anaesthetic, infiltrate the area subcutaneously now.

● Secure the skin adjacent to the vessel with your non-dominant thumb. Hold the cannula with your index finger pointing towards the needle, and enter the skin at an angle of about 45° (**11**). You will feel a pop as you enter the vein, and blood will 'flash-back' into the chamber at the top. Reduce the angle a little and use your non-dominant hand to advance the needle very slightly to check that the needle is in the vein. Hold the position of the cannula very still, and loosen the plastic sheath.

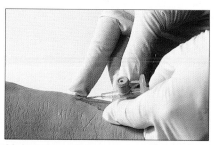

11 Inserting an intravenous cannula.

● Slowly and steadily advance the sheath along the line of the vein. Loosen the tourniquet. Apply pressure over the skin around the tip of the plastic sheath and remove the needle. Never attempt to replace the needle at this point as this could cause a piece of the plastic cannula to break off. Pick up the rubber spigot and place in the open end of the cannula, make a half-turn in a clockwise direction.

● Stick the cannula to the skin using a clear plastic dressing. Inject 2 ml of sterile saline through the cannula to keep it open.

Put all your instruments, cannulae, needles, vials, and disused ampoules in the cardboard tray and dispose of them at the nearest sharps bin. NEVER re-sheath needles. Dispose of any syringes in the yellow clinical waste bin.

Making up intravenous drugs

All drugs come with a data sheet that explains the essential facts about the preparation. Make sure you read this before you start.

Always check that you have the correct drug, correct dose, and that it is within date before injecting it.

You are often presented with a sealed vial of a drug, which may be in powder form. You may need to inject water into the vial to reconstitute the drug before you can aspirate it into the syringe (**12**). The description here will be of a vial of powdered antibiotic – this is the most commonly given intravenous preparation.

Giving an intravenous injection

Patients requiring several injections of an intravenous drug will frequently have a cannula *in situ*. Under these circumstances, you do not need to secure venous access as it is already available through the cannula. The cannula will have been sealed off with a rubber bung. When drawing up, you need also to prepare a syringe with a 21-gauge needle and 2 ml of sterile saline.

CHECK ALL DRUGS WITH YOUR ASSISTANT to ensure that the drug is correct, the dose is correct, and that the date is before the drug's expiry date.

Wipe the end of the rubber bung with a steret, aspirate and inject the drug directly into the bung. When this syringe is empty, inject the 2 ml of sterile saline to flush the cannula through. Leave the cannula *in situ* ready for the next injection.

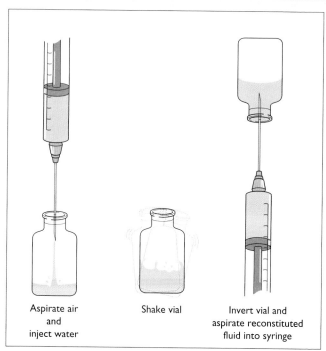

Aspirate air and inject water   Shake vial   Invert vial and aspirate reconstituted fluid into syringe

12 Making up intravenous (i.v.) drugs.

Preparing an intravenous injection

● Wash your hands before you begin, and open and clean the top of the vial, by flicking off the cover and wiping with an alcohol swab.

● Use a 10 ml sterile syringe and 21-gauge (green) needle. Aspirate 5–10 ml of sterile water into the syringe (**12**).

● Introduce the needle into the vial and aspirate 3–4 ml of air to create a vacuum. Allow the water to be sucked into the vial by this vacuum to dissolve the drug. Remove the needle and shake the vial vigorously to help drug dissolution.

● Reintroduce the needle and inject 3–4 ml of air; withdraw the needle to just inside the bung. Invert the vial and aspirate its contents into the syringe.

● Make the solution up to the required amount for injection by aspirating more sterile water.

Suturing technique

- Use the needle and the syringe of local anaesthetic. Warn the patient that it will sting. Inject beneath the skin edges from the apex of the wound at both ends. If the wound is large (more than 7 cm long), you may also need to infiltrate along the edges. Leave the anaesthetic to work for as long as possible, and check that it is working before proceeding.

- Open the suture material and clip the curved needle with the needle holder. The needle holders should be in the middle of the suture needle, and the suture needle half-way along the blades of the needle holders.

- Pick up the skin edge somewhere in the middle of the laceration with the fine-toothed forceps in your non-dominant hand (**13**). Hold the forceps as you would a pencil, with two teeth pointing up, and one tooth down. With the needle holder and suture in your dominant hand, pierce the skin at an angle of 90°. Pass under the wound in an arc, and push the needle through on the other side. If possible, do this in one movement; if this is not possible, come out in the middle of the wound, re-site the needle, and form another arc to reach the other side.

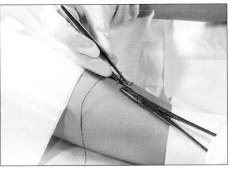

13 Pick up the edge of the skin with your fine-toothed forceps.

- You may need to use the toothed forceps to stabilize the skin and thus to help pull the needle through; then attach to the needle holder again. Pull the suture material through the wound until about 15 cm remains. Tie a surgical knot by looping the suture around the needle holder twice in a clockwise direction, and pulling the short end through, then twice in an anti-clockwise direction, and pulling the short end through again. Repeat the knot clockwise, then ask your assistant to cut at a distance of approximately 0.5 cm from the knot.

- Repeat the procedure for putting in sutures at regular intervals approximately 0.5 cm apart until the wound is held neatly together, and not gaping. Position your sutures specifically to hold the edges together well, but not too tight.

- Don't forget to cover the wound with a clean dry dressing and dispose of sharps carefully.

Suturing

Always introduce yourself and explain what you are going to do, and why. Outline how you will perform the procedure, and ask the patient if he/she has any questions. Make sure that you have the patient's verbal consent.

Before beginning the procedure, ensure that all the necessary equipment is there, and check the trolley. You need a suture pack, gloves, and suture material. You also require local anaesthetic and cleaning materials.

Remove your white coat, tuck in your tie if necessary, and wash your hands thoroughly at the beginning of the procedure. Open the suture pack without touching the inside of the paper. Ask your assistant to open a pair of the correct-sized gloves and let them fall onto the sterile area, i.e. the inside surface of the opened suture pack. Put on your gloves, touching their sterile outside surface as little as possible.

Arrange the equipment on the trolley so that everything is accessible, maintaining an aseptic technique. Ask your assistant to open a syringe and let it fall onto the sterile area; and to open a needle, connecting the green one to your syringe. Draw up the local anaesthetic. Put this down in your sterile area. Ask your assistant to fill the small pot with an appropriate cleaning fluid (normally chlorhexidine). Follow the procedure described for suturing technique.

Taking a history, examining a patient, and performing simple practical procedures are crucial to the role of a doctor. This chapter has outlined the overall process. The following chapters describe in detail the skills involved in the assessment of each system.

2 The cardiovascular system

Cardiac problems are among the most common causes of acute admission to hospital. They also form a large part of a general practitioner's workload. Patients are generally knowledgeable about the symptoms of heart disease, so it is frequently a cause for anxiety. It is essential that all medical practitioners are aware of the patterns of presentation of heart disease, and take the patient's symptoms seriously.

The most common problem relating to the cardiovascular system is coronary artery disease – and many patients die within the first few hours of a myocardial infarction, or of heart failure after several years of ill health. The incidence of coronary artery disease varies widely from country to country, but it has increased in industrialized countries throughout the 20th century. In some countries, such as Finland and the USA, rates have recently begun to decline, perhaps because of changes in diet and lifestyle. Japan and France have the lowest death rates per 100,000, and Finland and Scotland the highest.

Several factors influence predisposition to coronary artery disease – the 'coronary risk factors'. These are shown in Table 6, and should form the basis of questions put to patients presenting with chest pain.

Applied anatomy and physiology

All cardiac muscle has the intrinsic capacity for rhythmic excitation. The atria contain specialized fibres which are easily provoked into spontaneous rhythmic contraction, starting from the sino-atrial node. Ventricular muscle fibres can also contract on their own at a slow rhythm, but are normally excited through the specialized conducting tissues.

In isolation, the heart of a young adult will contract at an intrinsic rate about 110 beats/min (bpm). This intrinsic rate falls with age, and is about 80 bpm at the age of 70 years. The intrinsic rate is modified by the central nervous system, which can slow the heart by means of impulses transmitted in the

Table 6. Coronary risk factors

- Increasing age
- Male gender
- A family history of coronary artery disease
- Hypertension
- Obesity
- Smoking
- Diabetes
- Hyperlipidaemia
- A diet high in saturated fat

The healthy heart

The healthy heart obeys Starling's law, which states that the force of cardiac contraction increases with stroke volume, and so is dependent on cardiac filling.

• At a heart rate of 70 bpm in a young adult, each ventricle contains at the end of diastole about 120 ml of blood, 70 ml of which is expelled during systole. The **resting cardiac output** is therefore approximately 5 L/min.

• The force of cardiac contraction is continuously modified by the **ionic environment**, especially by the concentration of potassium and calcium in the blood.

• The **normal mean** pulmonary capillary pressure is probably only a few mmHg above mean alveolar pressure. Therefore, little extra pressure is needed to drive blood into the lungs.

• The **right ventricular pressure** is normally 20/0 mmHg and the **pulmonary artery pressure** about 20/8 mmHg, with a mean of 12 mmHg.

• The **mean left atrial pressure** is about 4 mmHg, the **left ventricular pressure** about 120/5 mmHg, and the **aortic pressure** 120/80 mmHg, with a mean of about 93 mmHg.

Most of the work of the heart is done by the left ventricle: the contraction of the left atrium makes only a small contribution to ventricular output.

vagus nerve, and speed it up by impulses in the sympathetic nerves and by adrenaline from the adrenal medulla. In a young adult, the heart is under predominantly vagal influence at rest and contracts at about 70 bpm. However, it may accelerate to 200 bpm or more during exertion. By the age of 60 years the maximum heart rate is about 170 bpm.

Any change in intrathoracic pressure has a large influence on venous return and hence on cardiac filling and cardiac output due to the small pressure gradient available to fill the heart. During a deep inspiration the intrathoracic pressure may be –25 mmHg, and during diastole most of this pressure is transmitted to the lax right ventricle, which sucks in blood. The diastolic volume of the right ventricle therefore increases and the ventricle has to raise a greater amount of blood to a greater effective pressure during deep inspiration.

Expiration, on the other hand, squeezes blood out of the lungs so that output from the left heart increases. Right ventricular contraction begins before left but finishes later, so that the pulmonary second heart sound (marking pulmonary valve closure) follows the aortic second sound. During inspiration, the increase in right ventricular volume prolongs the time taken for the right ventricle to expel its contents. Thus, the gap between the aortic and pulmonary second sound becomes wider.

Assessment and diagnosis of cardiovascular disease

Taking the history
Assessment of a patient with cardiovascular disease follows the same sequence and structure as for general history taking. The most frequent symptoms are chest pain and shortness of breath. These are both unpleasant and worrying symptoms, so it is important to recognize that the patient may be extremely anxious (and also possibly worried about dying). This may manifest itself in several ways.

The patient may appear angry, anxious, or reticent. It is the doctor's job to deal with these emotions effectively in order to take a full history. This is achieved by appearing confident, competent, and compassionate. Explore and reflect on their problems. Put the patient at ease before you start – remember that eye contact is important in establishing a rapport – and finally, make sure you listen (and look as if you are listening) to the patient's answers.

- Remember to start your history with an open question to encourage the patient to describe the symptoms more fully:
  'Tell me about your pain … How did it begin … What is it like?'
- Then move to more closed areas of enquiry such as:
  'What were you doing when it started … How long did it last?'

In general, it is better to encourage patients to describe the character of their symptoms in his/her own words.

The presenting complaint
Chest pain This is the main presenting symptom of angina or a myocardial infarction, although it can be caused by respiratory system problems or musculoskeletal problems. It is important to have a clear idea of what the pain is like. Cardiac pain is frequently described as crushing, heavy, or 'like a tight band around the chest'. Ask what the patient was doing when the pain came on, as angina is characteristically provoked by exercise. Find out if the pain goes anywhere else; cardiac pain often radiates to the left or both arms, or into the jaw. Ask about nausea, vomiting, and belching. Encourage the patient to estimate how long the pain lasted.

Breathlessness This is a common manifestation of cardiac disease, and it may be mentioned as a decrease in exercise tolerance or shortness of breath on climbing hills. Remember to ask how far the patient can walk before these symptoms appear:

- 'How far can you walk before feeling short of breath?'

Breathlessness may be at its worst at night.

Table 7. Important areas of enquiry
● **Chest pain**
● **Breathlessness**
● **Ankle swelling**
● **Syncope**
● **Palpitations**
● **Claudication**

Ask the patient whether he/she can lie flat, or how many pillows are required, and whether he/she is woken at night by shortness of breath:

- 'Can you lie flat? ... How many pillows do you use? ... Do you ever wake at night with shortness of breath?' ...

If so:

- 'What do you do?'

Patients often feel that they need to go to the window for some air. In association with breathlessness, patients may have other symptoms of heart failure, so enquire directly about swelling of the ankles:

- 'Have you noticed whether your ankles are swollen?'

Arrhythmias Patients with heart disease may suffer from arrhythmias, which may cause fainting (syncope) Ask:

- 'Have you ever had any blackouts? ... Tell me about them.'

Arrhythmias may also present, with palpitations – a feeling of awareness of the heartbeat. Most people understand this term. It is helpful to define whether the beats are 'regular or irregular', 'fast or slow', by asking the patient to tap out the beat of the palpitations on a table top.

Important areas of enquiry in cardiac patients are shown in **Table 7**. **Table 8** shows different kinds of chest pain.

Other important points from the history

Patients with ischaemic heart disease may also have symptoms of vascular disease in other parts of the body. The most common of these is intermittent claudication, a cramp-like pain in the legs on walking, which is relieved by rest. Ask the patient how far he/she can walk before having to stop, what stops him/her, how long it lasts, and whether he/she can continue walking after resting for a few minutes. Ask exactly where the claudication pain is located.

Past medical history

When asking about past medical history, it is important to enquire specifically about rheumatic fever, as this may predispose to valvular disease. The importance of this condition, however, is diminishing because it has become uncommon since the routine use of antibiotics for sore throats. Nevertheless, elderly patients, and those brought up in developing countries, may still have been affected. You must also ask about any history of hypertension and diabetes, or previous episodes of the cardiac symptoms outlined above. Enquire about previous chest pain and/or heart attacks.

Personal and social history

This is an important part of the history in cardiovascular disease, as it will show you the effect that the patient's symptoms have on his/her life. It also helps you to look for predisposing factors for cardiovascular disease in the patient's lifestyle.

Ask whether he/she takes any exercise, and what kind of activity he/she is able to perform before developing symptoms. This may overlap with the presenting complaint.

At this stage, you may feel that a sexual history is relevant. If the patient has had a straightforward myocardial infarction, it may not be important. However, under some circumstances it may be necessary to ask, for example, the older man whether he gets angina during intercourse, as this may be affecting his relationship with his partner.

Family history and treatment history

A family history of heart disease is a significant coronary risk factor. It is essential therefore to establish whether any close relatives have had chest pain or heart

Table 8. Examples of diferent kinds of chest pain

● *Angina*	Central tight pain on exercise, usual relieved by rest
● *Oesophageal pain/dyspepsia*	May be indistinguishable from angina
● *Pleuritic pain*	Sharp pain at the periphery of the chest, made worse by breathing
● *Pericarditic pain*	Like pleuritic pain, but relieved by leaning forward
● *Musculoskeletal pain*	May be related to previous unaccustomed exercise. Tender to touch, and may be worse on movement
● *Trauma*	History of excess alcohol or falls

attacks – or have suffered a sudden death. It is important to establish the age of the relative when these events occurred, as myocardial infarction runs in families.

Patients with cardiac conditions are often on multiple medications. Ask specifically if the patient has tried GTN (glyceryl trinitrate) and if it relieves pain, and how long it usually takes for relief to occur (GTN usually acts within five minutes for ischaemic chest pain). It is important to note down the medications and the dose, and also what has been tried in the past and any known reasons for stopping drugs. You can include tobacco and alcohol here. Ask whether the patient smokes; if the answer is 'no', then find out if he/she has ever smoked, and how much. Also ask why the patient gave up smoking. Follow exactly the same line of enquiry for alcohol.

A checklist for cardiovascular history taking is given in **Table 9**.

Table 9. Checklist for cardiovascular history taking
● General approach: introduce yourself, establish rapport. Remember eye contact
● Assess the present complaint and its history (previous attacks, nature of pain, etc.). Don't forget the coronary risk factors
● Ask about past medical history, particularly in relation to heart disease
● Ask about smoking/drinking/drugs
● Ask about social history, e.g. how many stairs in the home?
● Ask about family history, does anyone have heart disease or chest pain?
● Systematic enquiry
Finally– LISTEN TO THE ANSWERS!

Examination of the patient

In order to perform a thorough cardiovascular examination, the patient should be comfortable and relaxed. Make sure that the room is not too cold. First, look at the patient's hands, check the neck, pulses and blood pressure, then follow the scheme: inspection, palpation, auscultation.

General observation

Begin the examination with an assessment of the patient's general condition.

Does he/she look well or ill – are they comfortable or short of breath at rest?

Does he/she have central cyanosis? Take the body temperature.

Then, look at the patient's hands. In

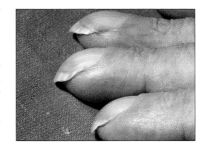

14 Finger clubbing.

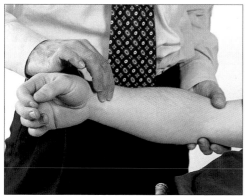

15 Feeling the radial pulse.

the cardiovascular system you are looking for peripheral cyanosis, clubbing (**14**), and splinter haemorrhages. Next look for anaemia in the conjunctiva, and re-check for central cyanosis.

Arterial pulses

The radial pulse should be palpated, as illustrated (**15**). The pulse should be confirmed as being equal and synchronous in both wrists with the rate, rhythm, volume, and character noted.

The radial pulse is usually counted over 15 seconds, and the rate (bpm) calculated. The rhythm of the pulse should be regular, apart from normal inspiratory speeding (sinus arrhythmia). You should ask yourself the following questions if the pulse is irregular:

- Is the pulse basically regular but with occasional irregularities (extra beats, or pauses)? This suggests the presence of ectopic beats (i.e. beats arising from some focus other than the sinoatrial node). Ectopic beats may arise either in the ventricle or at a supraventricular site (atrium or atrioventricular node). If they are ventricular in origin, they are usually followed by a compensatory pause.
- Is the pulse totally irregular both in timing and volume? This suggests atrial fibrillation. It sometimes may be difficult to analyse the cardiac rhythm simply by feeling the pulse – the rhythm may be resolved by auscultation. You may hear the terms 'irregular irregular pulse' or 'regular irregular pulse'. This is confusing terminology – it is easier to state that a pulse is either 'irregular' or 'regular'.

The volume of the pulse should be checked next – does the amplitude feel small or large? A small-volume pulse suggests a low stroke volume and reduced

Pulses and their identification

- The **brachial pulse** (**21**) is best felt in the patient's right arm by applying the fingers or thumb of your right hand to the front of the elbow just medial to the biceps tendon, with the fingers supporting the back of the elbow.

- The **carotid pulse** (**17**) is best felt on the patient's right side: locate the mid-point of the anterior border of the sternomastoid muscle with the fingers or thumb of your left hand (this is often the site of a skin crease) and press firmly backwards. Do not feel both carotid pulses at the same time, as you will temporarily obstruct the cerebral blood flow, especially in the elderly. Three main abnormalities are slow rising, collapsing, and bisferiens.

cardiac output, while a large-volume pulse may signify a large left ventricular stroke volume. Avoid the terms 'a weak' or 'a strong' pulse, particularly in front of patients.

The character of the pulse refers to the shape of the pulse wave. This is better assessed at the brachial pulse or, more particularly, at the carotid because of its size and its proximity to the heart. The pulse wave is greatly altered by transmission through the arterial tree, and certain abnormalities may be much more easily detected at one site rather than another.

Pulsus paradoxus is the term applied when the pulse is felt to become much reduced in volume on inspiration. During the respiratory cycle, the intrathoracic pressure becomes more negative as the lungs expand during inspiration. As a direct result, blood pools in the pulmonary vessels and the filling of the left ventricle is reduced (*see* 'Physiology', page 42). While this pressure difference may be palpated, it is usually quantified by measuring the difference in systolic blood pressure occurring between inspiration and expiration. This is done by deflating the sphygmomanometer cuff very slowly and listening to the sounds appearing and disappearing as the level of mercury falls.

This reduction of left ventricular stroke volume can be exaggerated, as in pericardial tamponade or asthma, and is detectable both by palpating the peripheral pulses or when measuring the blood pressure. The pulse volume feels less on inspiration and greater on expiration (the 'paradox').

Peripheral arterial pulse examination
The femoral pulses are best examined with the patient undressed and lying flat. The examiner should firmly apply the thumb just below the mid-inguinal point(**16**). Check that the radial pulses are synchronous with the femoral pulse – in coarctation of the aorta the pulse is both reduced in volume and appreciably delayed compared with the radial pulse.

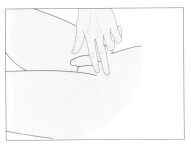

16 Feeling the femoral pulse.

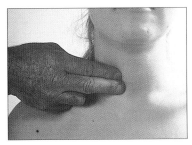

17 Feeling the carotid pulse.

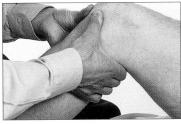

18 Feeling the popliteal pulse.

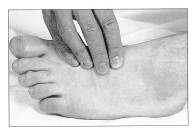

19 Feeling the dorsalis pedis pulse.

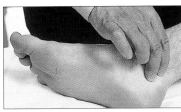

20 Feeling the tibialis posterior pulse.

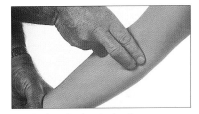

21 Feeling the brachial pulse.

The volume of the pulse should be noted and the stethoscope used to listen for a bruit over where the pulse is felt in the groin. The popliteal pulses lie deep within the popliteal fossa and are best felt by compressing them against the posterior surface of the distal end of the femur with the fingertips of both hands (18). The patient should be lying flat with the knee flexed. The positions of the dorsalis pedis and tibialis posterior are shown (19, 20), as well as the brachial pulse.(21)

Jugular venous pressure
In assessing the jugular venous pressure (JVP), the cervical veins form a blood-filled manometer connected to the right atrium and, as such, can be used at the

Monitoring the JVP

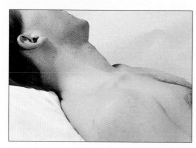

22 Inspect the JVP with the patient resting at an angle of 45°.

The internal jugular vein should be inspected with the patient resting on a pillow at 45° (**22**). It is sometimes helpful to direct a light onto the root of the neck. Venous pulsations can be distinguished from arterial pulsations in the neck in the following way:
- They are usually abolished by gentle pressure on the veins at the root of the neck.
- They often vary with respiration and can be made to rise by firm pressure over the upper abdomen.
- A rapid flickering and inward movement is the usual component, whereas arterial pulsations are typically outward pulses.

bedside to measure the mean right atrial pressure (central venous pressure, CVP). In addition, they can provide information about the wave form in the right atrium.

Whenever possible, the right internal jugular vein is used for the assessment because it is in direct communication with the superior vena cava (SVC) and the right atrium – pressure in the left internal jugular vein may be raised spuriously as a consequence of partial obstruction of the innominate vein by the arch of the aorta. The observation of the JVP is a difficult skill, and so has been covered in some detail here. It is easier to see if you know what you are looking for!

The mean level of the venous pressure should be measured with reference to the sternal angle (**23**). Generally, it is at the level of the angle – if it is ≥2 cm above this with the patient at 45°, the pressure is definitely raised (**24**). A raised JVP reflects a raised end-diastolic pressure in the right ventricle. If the JVP is grossly elevated, but the cervical veins show no pulsation, then obstruction to the SVC should be suspected.

It is often possible to identify the 'a' and 'v' waves of the normal venous pulse. The waves of the venous pulse are most easily identified by timing them

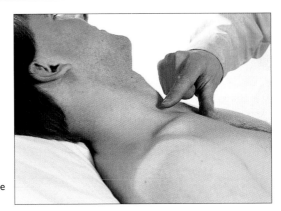

23 Measure venous pressure with reference to the sternal angle.

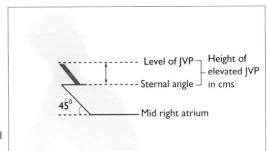

24 The level of the JVP in relation to the sternal angle.

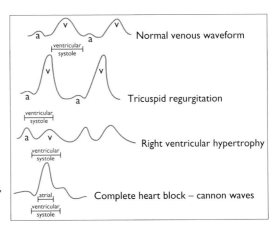

25 Venous waveforms seen in the JVP in a normal tricuspid regurgitation, right ventricular hypertrophy, and complete heart block.

against the carotid pulse, which provides a convenient indication of ventricular systole. They may occur either just before the carotid pulse = 'a' waves (pre-systole) or approximately with the carotid = 'v' wave (systole) (25).

Abnormally large 'a' waves are associated with right ventricular hypertrophy and tricuspid stenosis. The 'a' wave is absent in atrial fibrillation.

Abnormally large systolic 'v' waves may be caused by tricuspid regurgitation with reflux of blood during systole from the right ventricle.

Cannon wave results from contraction of the atrium against a closed tricuspid valve in complete heart block.

Measuring the blood pressure

Blood pressure is recorded by writing the systolic pressure over the diastolic pressure with some notation of the position of the patient (Table 10). A normal blood pressure is approximately as shown.

Table 10. Blood pressure	
$^{120}/_{80}$	**Lying**
$^{115}/_{80}$	**Standing**

Inspection of the precordium

Inspection of the precordium is usually unhelpful – however, the apex beat may not be visible. It is also important to note any scars such as that of a mitral valvotomy under the left breast, or a sternal split for a valve replacement or coronary artery bypass grafts.

Measuring the blood pressure

The sphygmomanometer cuff should be smoothly applied around the unclothed upper arm, with the left hand supporting the patient's arm. If the arm is exceptionally thick or thin (e.g. extreme obesity, or in children), the standard cuff will give inaccurate readings and one appropriate for the arm size must be used. Modern cuffs use Velcro to secure them. Make sure you put it on with the airbag underneath, or the cuff will come apart when you blow it up (**26**).

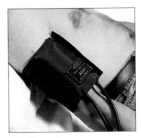

26 The sphygmomanometer.

● Once the cuff is in position, close the screw valve and pump it up to a level above your estimation of the blood pressure (approximately 130 mmHg).

● As the pressure in the sphygmomanometer cuff increases above the systolic pressure in the brachial artery, the artery is compressed and the radial pulse becomes impalpable.

● As the pressure in the cuff is then gradually lowered, blood can force its way past the obstruction for part of the cardiac cycle, creating sounds which can be heard with the diaphragm of the stethoscope placed over the brachial artery (Korotkoff sounds). As the pressure in the cuff is further lowered, the Korotkoff sounds become louder and more ringing in nature, and then suddenly become muffled. Very shortly afterwards, the sounds usually disappear altogether.

● The point where you first hear the sound is the systolic measurement, and it is the point of disappearance which is conventionally used to measure the diastolic blood pressure (phase 5). The pressure always varies to some extent, so it is acceptable to measure it and round it off to the nearest 5 mmHg.

● It is good practice to check the systolic pressure approximately by palpation of the radial artery before applying the stethoscope; this helps you to confirm the reading you hear. When there is considerable beat-to-beat variation in pressure (as in atrial fibrillation), the average level of the systolic and diastolic pressure must be judged by ear.

● When the blood pressure is seriously reduced and it is difficult to hear the Korotkoff sounds, it may be easier to measure the systolic blood pressure by palpation, noting the level at which the pulse is felt first as the cuff is deflated – diastolic pressure cannot be recorded satisfactorily by palpation.

Palpation of the precordium

The apex beat is the point furthest to the left and downwards at which a definite cardiac impulse is felt; this should be located by palpation using the flat of the hand and the fingertips with the patient lying at 45°. It normally lies within the 5th intercostal space and within the mid-clavicular line. If the apex beat is felt further out, it usually means there is enlargement of one or both ventricles or displacement of the heart to the left by chest deformity or disease of the lungs.

Now assess the quality of the impulse. A forceful apex beat usually indicates increased cardiac output: in left ventricular hypertrophy the apex beat is distinctive with a sustained and forceful heave compared with the usual short, sharp impulse. In mitral stenosis, the apex beat is often described as tapping – this is due partly to displacement of the left ventricle nearer to the examining hand by an enlarged left ventricle, and partly due to a palpable first heart sound.

Right ventricular hypertrophy is detected by firm pressure with the flat of your hand over the left sternal edge. In adults, the normal right ventricle does not produce a definite impulse, while in right ventricular hypertrophy a definite parasternal heave may be felt. Occasionally, the right ventricle may enlarge anteriorly to replace the left ventricle in forming the apex of the heart. It is important to confirm the impulse felt by using bimanual examination placing the flat of left hand against the sternal border with the right hand feeling the apical impulse – two separate impulses are detectable where both ventricles are enlarged. During palpation of the precordium thrills may be felt: these are the low-frequency components of loud murmurs which are more easily confirmed after auscultation.

Percussion

In the examination of the cardiovascular system, it is not usually helpful to percuss over the precordium, except to locate the position of the mediastinum. This is useful in cases where it may be displaced, e.g. chronic airflow limitation, or right lung collapse. If you do not suspect mediastinal shift from the history or the tracheal position, do not percuss the position of the mediastinum.

Auscultation

The stethoscope has two principal functions: to transmit sounds from the chest wall with exclusion of extraneous noises, and to emphasize sounds of certain frequencies. The bell of the stethoscope is best for listening to low-pitched sounds, whereas the diaphragm filters out low-pitched sounds and accentuates high-pitched ones. You should initially listen with the bell and diaphragm at the apex (**27**) for the low-pitched diastolic murmur of mitral stenosis, and the pan-systolic murmur of mitral regurgitation. Then, using the diaphragm, listen over the classical areas shown in **28**. These are the left sternal edge (for tricuspid murmurs) (**29**), the left second interspace (for pulmonary murmurs) (**30**), and the right second interspace (for aortic murmurs) (**31**).

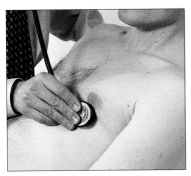

27 Listen with the bell at the apex.

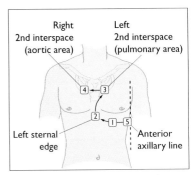

Right
2nd interspace
(aortic area)

Left
2nd interspace
(pulmonary area)

Left sternal
edge

Anterior
axillary line

28 Classic areas for listening to heart sounds: Apex (1), Left sternal edge (2), Left second interspace (3), Right second interspace (4).

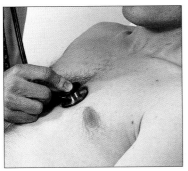

29 Listening at the left sternal edge.

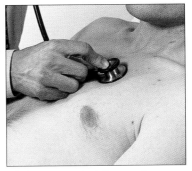

30 Listening at the left second interspace.

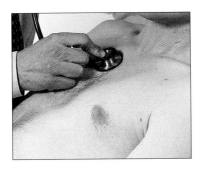

31 Listening at the right second interspace.

Heart sounds

It is impossible to listen critically to more than one sound at any one time, so try to train yourself to listen for single components of the heart sounds.

First heart sound This is produced mainly by the mitral and tricuspid valve closure, and caused by the sudden tensing of the valve as it halts after ballooning back into the atrium at the beginning of systole. The loudness of the mitral closure, which is normally the main component of the first heart sound, depends on the force with which it is thrust back into the atrium, and this may be altered, for example in mitral stenosis. The length of the interval between atrial and ventricular systole also influences the loudness of the first heart sound. The sound is loudest when the PR interval is short (see **38** page 63).

Second heart sound This is produced by closure of the aortic and pulmonary valves. If the valve cusps lose their mobility, as in calcific aortic stenosis, the sound produced at the affected valve is reduced and may be completely lost. The second heart sound splits into two components during inspiration, and these come together in expiration. This physiological splitting is due to minor changes in the stroke volume of the left and right ventricles during the normal respiratory cycle. During inspiration, the venous return to the right side of the heart is increased, thus increasing the right ventricular stroke volume and delaying closure of the pulmonary valve. At the same time, pooling of the blood in the pulmonary veins reduces the filling of the left ventricle and makes aortic valve closure slightly earlier compared with expiration. This process is reversed in expiration (**32**). The split may be widened by other factors which delay right ventricular contraction: examples are listed in **33**.

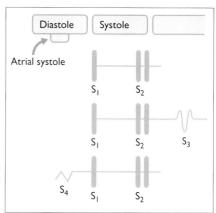

32 The relationship between heart sounds and diastole and systole: the lower portion of the figure denotes the usual way to record heart sounds.

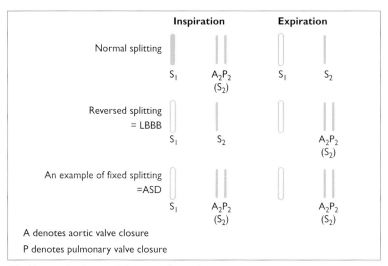

33 Abnormal splitting of the second sound.

Third and fourth heart sounds A third heart sound is usually a low-frequency sound best heard with the bell, and occurring just after the second heart sound. It is caused by the sudden distension of the ventricle at the end of the rapid filling phase in early diastole. A soft third heart sound may be heard at the apex in most normal children and adults less than 30 years of age: in older people it is abnormal and signifies unusually abrupt filling of the ventricle. This may arise from an abnormally large stroke volume or from increased ventricular filling pressure due to left ventricular failure.

A fourth heart sound is also a low-frequency sound: it is best heard immediately before the first heart sound and signifies that atrial systole is abnormally forceful. The presence of an atrial (fourth) sound implies that the end-diastolic pressure is raised in the ventricle concerned, e.g. the left ventricle in systemic hypertension.

Gallop rhythm A gallop rhythm means that there are three heart sounds to the cycle, and that the extra one is either a third sound or an atrial (fourth) sound. The noises heard sound rather like Kentucky ('ken-tuc-kee'). At rapid heart rates, the third heart sound and atrial sounds may coincide and a summation gallop is then heard – the noise suggests Tennessee ('ten-nes-see'). In clinical practice, this suggests impaired ventricular function.

The usual way to record heart sounds is shown in **33**.

Factors that may cause murmurs

- Increased velocity of flow.
- Localized constriction of the lumen through which the blood is flowing, with turbulence developing where the lumen widens out again.
- Roughening of a surface past which blood is flowing (e.g. atheromatous plaque).
- Decreased viscosity of blood.

Murmurs

Cardiac murmurs result either from abnormal turbulence of blood flow or from vibrations in structures adjacent to an area of turbulent flow. Factors favouring the development of turbulence giving rise to murmurs are shown above. Commonly, more than one of these factors is involved.

When a murmur is heard it is essential to note:

- The site of maximum intensity and the direction of radiation.
- The timing of the murmur.
- The loudness.
- The quality – is it high- or low-pitched, or musical?
- The presence or absence of a palpable thrill.

Timing of the murmur A murmur produced at a particular valve has a characteristic timing, as it may only occur when there is a pressure gradient across the valve. Timing of the murmur is of great help in its recognition. In timing it is important to decide whether the murmur occurs in systole or diastole – if there is doubt, the murmur should be timed against the carotid pulse. The timing of the murmur is then analysed in relation to the heart sounds. The usual sites and radiation of the common cardiac murmurs are shown in **34**.

Systolic murmurs Systolic murmurs are due to one of three factors:

1 Pansystolic murmur: leakage of blood through a valve structure which is usually closed during systole. The intensity of the murmur is therefore very similar throughout the length of systole.

2. Ejection systolic murmur: the flow through a valve which is normally open in systole but which has become abnormally narrowed. The murmur typically starts quietly, rises to a crescendo mid-systole, and then becomes quiet towards the end of systole.

3 Increased blood flow through a normal valve, physiological flow murmur – the character is identical to that heard in ejection systolic murmur.

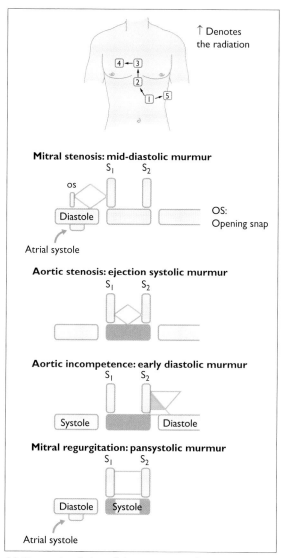

34 Sites and radiation of the common cardiac murmurs.

Identifying diastolic murmurs

● An **early diastolic murmur** is nearly always due to incompetence of either the aortic or pulmonary valve. It is maximum at the beginning of diastole when aortic or pulmonary pressure is highest, and rapidly becomes quieter as pressure falls. The murmur of aortic incompetence can be amplified by getting the patient to sit forward, placing the diaphragm of the stethoscope over the left sternal edge, and then asking the patient to hold his/her breath at the end of expiration.

● A **mid-diastolic murmur** is usually due to blood flow through a narrowed mitral or tricuspid valve, and the murmur is characteristically low-pitched and 'rumbling', and audible throughout the remainder of diastole. A mid-diastolic murmur may be made more obvious by having the patient lie on the left side, and for you to listen with the bell of the stethoscope over the apex.

Diastolic murmurs Diastolic murmurs can be divided into early diastolic and mid-diastolic (see above). A diagrammatic explanation for the murmurs associated with mitral stenosis, mitral incompetence, aortic stenosis, and aortic incompetence is shown in **34**.

Examination of the chest and ankles It is important to sit the patient forward at the end of the examination of the cardiovascular system to examine the lung bases for crackles and/or a pleural effusion. The ankles must also be examined for evidence of pitting oedema – press firmly over the tibia, and see whether an indentation remains after the finger is removed.

Illustrated physical signs

Left ventricular failure or pulmonary oedema is characterized by shadowing on the chest X-ray in a bat's wing distribution (**35**).

Peripheral oedema (**36**) is also a sign of predominantly right-sided heart failure. There may be indentation after the examiner has removed his/her finger from the surface of the tibia after applying mild pressure.

A patient with ischaemic heart disease may have an *arcus senilis*, suggesting a chronically high level of plasma cholesterol (**37**).

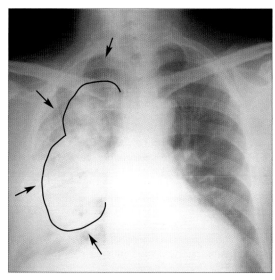

35 Pulmonary oedema on a chest X-ray (a bat's wing), more pronounced on the right.

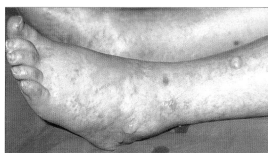

36 Peripheral oedema with blistering.

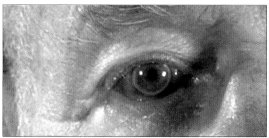

37 *Arcus senilis* in a patient with ischaemic heart disease.

Table 11. Normal cardiovascular examination	
● *Hands and face*	No cyanosis, pallor, clubbing, etc.
● *Pulses*	Radial, brachial, carotid: normal character, sinus rhythm, normal volume rate 60–90 bpm. No audible bruits over
● *JVP*	Visible at the sternal angle or 2 cm above with visible 'a' and 'v' waves
● *Apex beat*	At the 5th intercostal space, mid-clavicular line. No thrills or heaves
● *Heart sounds*	Normal S_1 followed by physiologically split S_2 and no added sounds
● *Lung bases*	No crackles
● *Ankles*	No ankle oedema. No sacral oedema
● *Blood pressure*	Do not forget to check the blood pressure yourself. Normal systolic pressure usually between 100–150 mmHg, but dependent upon the person's age. Normal diastolic pressure usually 70–90 mmHg, but dependent upon the person's age

The examination findings in a normal patient are shown in **Table 11**. Important aspects of care of the cardiovascular patient are shown in **Table 12**.

Therapeutic and interventional skills

An ECG and a chest X-ray are two important investigations which are required to complete the clinical assessment of the cardiovascular system.

The ECG

The ECG must be used as part of the diagnostic process alongside the clinical history. If the history is suggestive of a myocardial infarction (MI), the patient should be treated as if s/he is having an infarct, even if the ECG is normal. A patient with chest pain and a normal ECG may be in the very early stages of a MI; this is when there is the greatest risk of death. In a patient with chest pain it may be necessary for the ECG to be repeated later in the day to see if there have been any changes. The ECG pattern is recorded in a single lead during one heartbeat, and called an ECG complex; its components are shown in **38**. (An example of the evolution of the changes in an ECG during a myocardial infarction are shown in **39**.)

Table 12. Care of the patient with cardiovascular disease

- Appreciate the patient's anxiety
- Bed rest – cardiac bed (resting until pain-free in myocardial infarction/angina)
- Keep them sitting up in bed at 45° or on at least 3–4 pillows (to prevent dyspnoea)
- No added salt in diet (to minimize water retention)
- Oxygen always available (to maximize tissue oxygenation)
- Think about anticoagulation (many patients may require this)
- Cardiac monitoring may be necessary (to check arrhythmias)
- May need daily weight check if in heart failure (best indication of fluid retention)
- Frequent ECG monitoring

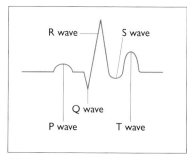

38 ECG pattern of a single heartbeat in a single lead. P = atrial depolarization; QRS = ventricular depolarization; T = repolarization.

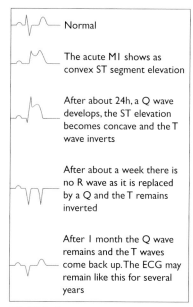

Normal

The acute MI shows as convex ST segment elevation

After about 24h, a Q wave develops, the ST elevation becomes concave and the T wave inverts

After about a week there is no R wave as it is replaced by a Q and the T remains inverted

After 1 month the Q wave remains and the T waves come back up. The ECG may remain like this for several years

39 ECG changes over time following a myocardial infarction. Note: it is possible to tell where the MI is located by noting which leads show the features most clearly – e.g. II, III, and AVF reflect inferior damage.

Table 13. The ECG machine

● *Four limb leads*	Right arm	RED
	Left arm	YELLOW
	Right leg	GREEN
	Left leg	BLACK
● *One chest lead*	Six sticky or suction electrodes	
● *Electrode jelly*	(alcohol swabs will do)	

Performing an ECG

Before taking the ECG recorder to the patient, make sure you have all the parts. These are shown in **Table 13**. Explain the procedure to the patient, i.e. 'I am going to do an electrical recording of your heart; it is not painful, and should only take a couple of minutes'. Check that the patient agrees (gives verbal consent) to the tracing.

● A standard 12-lead machine will perform the ECG at one time, so attach all limb and chest leads before taking the trace. If you are using a single-channel machine (sometimes the only kind available on the wards), record from the limb leads first, and then attach and record the chest leads one by one.

● The limb leads are usually labelled, and relate to a diagram drawn on the side of the ECG machine. If not, use the colour code shown in **Table 13**. Attach the arm leads to the patient's wrists. Contact is better in hairless areas, i.e. the inner aspect of the forearm and the outer aspect of the leg, just above the ankle. The positions of the chest leads are shown in **40** and **Table 14**.

● Once you have the machine correctly wired, make sure it is properly calibrated by keeping the dial on 0, with the paper running, and press the 1 mV marker. The height of the mark on the trace should be 10 small squares. Leads I, II, III, AVR, AVL, and AVF can then be measured by switching to record either for individual leads, or together in a 12-lead machine.

● Once this is complete (or concurrently in a multichannel machine), you can proceed to recording the chest or V leads, from the positions shown in **Table 14**.

● When the trace is complete, record the patient's name, and the date and time of the trace, and label the trace from each lead if this has not been done automatically. A photograph of a normal trace is shown in **41**, and one in a patient suffering an acute MI in **42**.

Table 14. Position of the chest (V) leads

V1	Fourth intercostal space, right of the sternum
V2	Fourth intercostal space, left of the sternum
V3	Between V2 and V4
V4	Left fifth intercostal space in the mid clavicular line
V5	Anterior axillary line level with V4
V6	Mid axillary line, level with V4

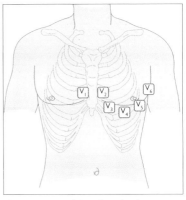

40 Positions of the chest leads.

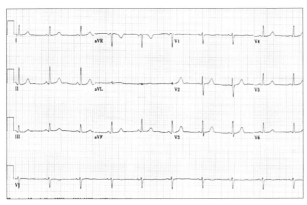

41 A normal 12-lead ECG.

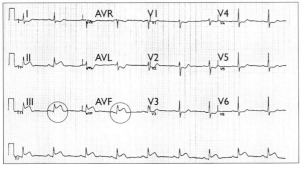

42 The ECG changes during an acute inferior myocardial infarct. Note the concave ST segment elevation (circles).

Table 15. ECG interpretation

Rate	Count the number of 5-mm squares between the R waves, and divide into 300 to give the beats per minute (bpm)
Rhythm	Is it regular; are P waves followed by QRS?
Axis	Look at two perpendicular leads, e.g. I and AVF, and count the number of squares – the tallest R wave indicates the main line of depolarization (axis)
Complexes	The P wave, and PR interval The QRS complex The T wave

Interpretation of the ECG When examining the trace, remember that the different leads of the ECG are looking at the heart from different directions. These directions are in a sagittal plane for the limb leads, and a coronal plane for the V leads (43). This allows you to work out where an abnormality is coming from. If the trace is abnormal in leads II, III, and AVF, the problem is inferior, as in 39; if the trace is abnormal in leads I, AVL, and V6, the problem is lateral, and on the left.

It is useful to develop a system for interpreting the trace to ensure nothing is overlooked. A practical system is outlined in **Table 15** (above).

In addition to the sequential interpretation of an ECG, it is useful to be able to recognize some common patterns. A selection of these is illustrated below (44–50).

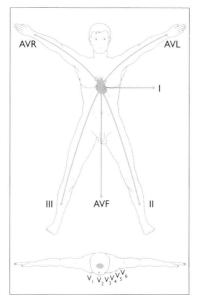

43 The ECG leads looking at the heart from different directions.

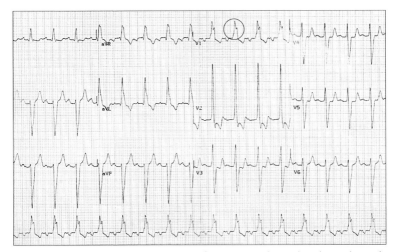

44 Right bundle branch block. Note the RSR pattern with a widened complex and inverted T wave in V1.

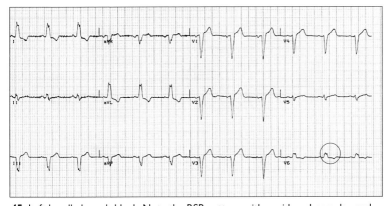

45 Left bundle branch block. Note the RSR pattern with a widened complex and inverted T wave in V5–6.

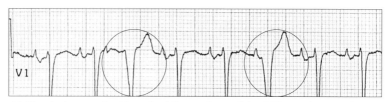

46 Ventricular ectopics. Note the different shape of the QRS complexes in the affected beats.

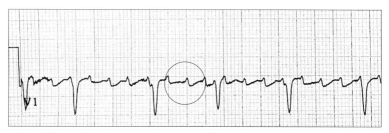

47 Atrial flutter. Note the sawtooth pattern with irregular ventricular complexes.

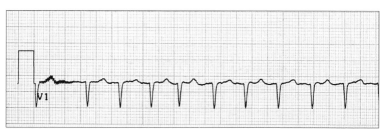

48 Atrial fibrillation (AF). Note the irregular rhythm and the absence of clear P waves.

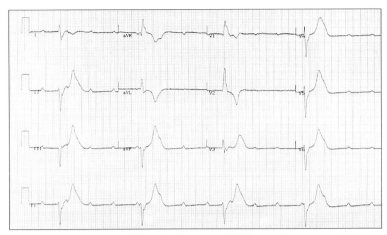

49 Complete heart block. Note the P waves and QRS complexes are regular but do not relate to each other.

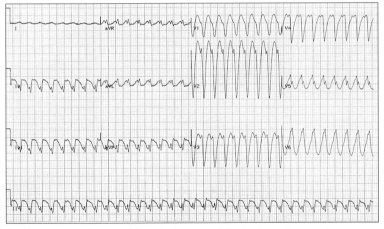

50 Ventricular tachycardia. Note the fast rate with wide irregular complexes.

Key laboratory tests

In angina and the early stages of a MI, the haemoglobin and white blood cells are normal. As an infarction evolves, there may be a neutrophil leukocytosis, though this settles as the condition settles.

Cardiac enzymes   The cardiac enzymes are used to confirm a suspected diagnosis of a myocardial infarction. The enzymes reflect death of cardiac muscle cells. The two enzymes most commonly measured are creatine kinase (CK) and aspartate transaminase (AST). CK is specific for cardiac muscle, and rises within a few hours of an infarct. A raised AST can be detected within 12–24 hours after infarction, and will return to normal 48–72 hours later, although this gives supportive evidence. The enzyme is also found in liver and lung, and so is less specific. A more specific test, Troponin, is now available in most hospitals.

Chest X-ray   A good quality postero-anterior (PA) X-ray of the chest will provide considerable information about both the heart and lung fields. The cardiac silhouette in the posteroanterior view normally appears as shown in **51**.

The right border of the normal cardiac shadow consists of:

- Slightly curved portion = outer edge of the superior vena cava with ascending aorta.
- A more convex portion = outer border of the right atrium, the lower margin of which lies at the diaphragm.

The left border of the cardiac shadow comprizes:

- A prominent knuckle produced by the arch of the aorta as it passes backwards.
- A straighter line of the pulmonary artery.
- Left atrial appendage.
- Wide sweep of the left ventricle, ending at the apex where it rests on the diaphragm.

The site of the heart as a whole can be assessed by measuring the cardiothoracic index – the ratio of the maximum width of the cardiac silhouette to the maximum width of the thorax, measured from rib to rib (**51**). The ratio can only be assessed on a postero-anterior film. In normal circumstances it is less than 50%. Enlargement of the left ventricle and right atrium are usually easily identified. Enlargement of the left atrium is often seen as an area of added density within the cardiac outline.

Key features of common cardiovascular conditions are depicted in **52–57**.

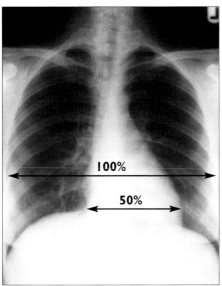

51 A normal PA chest X-ray.

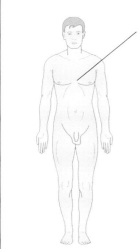

History
Crushing chest pain generally relieved by rest in angina but not in myocardial infarction

Examination findings
The patient may be in pain

There is usually little to find but look for evidence of risk factors – nicotine stains, xanthelasma, corneal arcus

Always measure the blood pressure and examine the fundi for hypertensive changes

There may be evidence of peripheral vascular disease

Examine the peripheral pulses

52 Ischaemic heart disease.

History

Symptoms of biventricular (congestive) cardiac failure. May present acutely as LVF

Examination findings

JVP raised in biventricular failure and tricuspid incompetence

Left parasternal heave. Displaced apex beat towards the axilla

Pansystolic murmur radiates to the axilla

Fine basal crepitations in LVF

Enlarged liver in biventricular failure; may be pulsatile if asociated tricuspid regurgitation

53 Mitral incompetence.

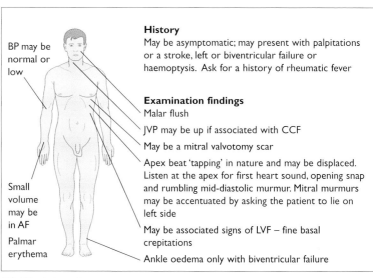

BP may be normal or low

History

May be asymptomatic; may present with palpitations or a stroke, left or biventricular failure or haemoptysis. Ask for a history of rheumatic fever

Examination findings

Malar flush

JVP may be up if associated with CCF

May be a mitral valvotomy scar

Apex beat 'tapping' in nature and may be displaced. Listen at the apex for first heart sound, opening snap and rumbling mid-diastolic murmur. Mitral murmurs may be accentuated by asking the patient to lie on left side

Small volume may be in AF

Palmar erythema

May be associated signs of LVF – fine basal crepitations

Ankle oedema only with biventricular failure

54 Mitral stenosis.

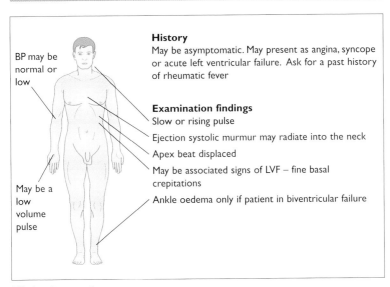

BP may be normal or low

History
May be asymptomatic. May present as angina, syncope or acute left ventricular failure. Ask for a past history of rheumatic fever

Examination findings
Slow or rising pulse

Ejection systolic murmur may radiate into the neck

Apex beat displaced

May be associated signs of LVF – fine basal crepitations

Ankle oedema only if patient in biventricular failure

May be a low volume pulse

55 Aortic stenosis.

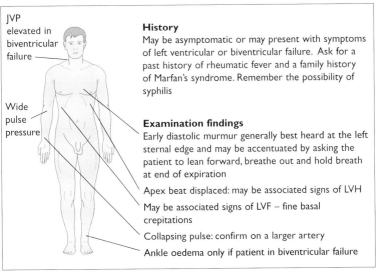

JVP elevated in biventricular failure

Wide pulse pressure

History
May be asymptomatic or may present with symptoms of left ventricular or biventricular failure. Ask for a past history of rheumatic fever and a family history of Marfan's syndrome. Remember the possibility of syphilis

Examination findings
Early diastolic murmur generally best heard at the left sternal edge and may be accentuated by asking the patient to lean forward, breathe out and hold breath at end of expiration

Apex beat displaced: may be associated signs of LVH

May be associated signs of LVF – fine basal crepitations

Collapsing pulse: confirm on a larger artery

Ankle oedema only if patient in biventricular failure

56 Aortic incompetence.

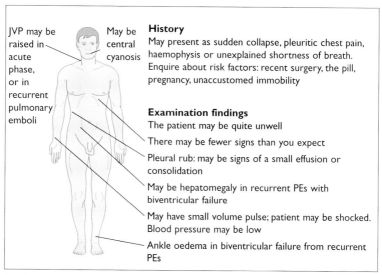

JVP may be raised in acute phase, or in recurrent pulmonary emboli

May be central cyanosis

History
May present as sudden collapse, pleuritic chest pain, haemophysis or unexplained shortness of breath. Enquire about risk factors: recent surgery, the pill, pregnancy, unaccustomed immobility

Examination findings
The patient may be quite unwell

There may be fewer signs than you expect

Pleural rub: may be signs of a small effusion or consolidation

May be hepatomegaly in recurrent PEs with biventricular failure

May have small volume pulse; patient may be shocked. Blood pressure may be low

Ankle oedema in biventricular failure from recurrent PEs

57 Pulmonary emboli.

Varicose veins and venous insufficiency

Applied anatomy and physiology of the venous system in the legs

The anatomy of the venous system in the legs is shown in 58. Numerous perforating veins link the superficial veins to the deep system, especially in the calf. In addition to venae commitantes running with the three principal calf arteries, the deep system includes large, thin-walled venous sinusoids lying between the calf muscles. These are an important component of the calf muscle pump. When the calf muscles contract, the deep veins are compressed and blood is propelled towards the heart. When the muscles relax, low pressure in the deep system encourages blood to move from superficial to deep via the perforating veins. Activity in the calf muscle pump is capable of reducing resting blood pressure in foot veins from about 100 mmHg during standing to about 20 mmHg on exercise.

The calf muscle pump becomes less effective if varicosity and valvular incompetence lead to retrograde flow in superficial veins. It becomes markedly

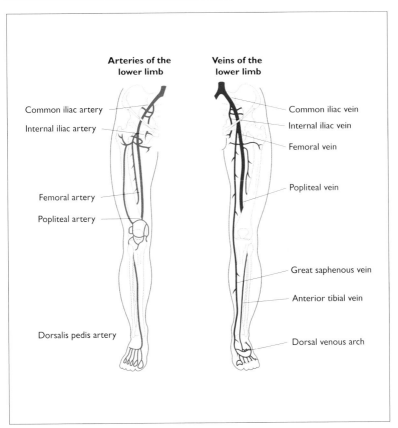

Arteries of the lower limb

Common iliac artery
Internal iliac artery
Femoral artery
Popliteal artery
Dorsalis pedis artery

Veins of the lower limb

Common iliac vein
Internal iliac vein
Femoral vein
Popliteal vein
Great saphenous vein
Anterior tibial vein
Dorsal venous arch

58 The venous system of the legs.

less effective if the deep venous valves are incompetent, as blood pumped proximally tends to flow back down to the calf when the muscles relax (reflux). Perforator vein incompetence may worsen the situation further. It should be noted, however, that the calf muscle pump is composed of both venous and muscular elements and failure of either will give rise to chronic venous hypertension. Severe immobility (due to paresis, arthritis, obesity, and other causes) may thus result in chronic venous insufficiency.

Assessment and diagnosis of venous disorders

Taking the history
Presenting complaint

A patient with varicose veins (59) may complain of the appearance of his/her legs, of aching legs, or may have suffered with ulceration (60), thrombophlebitis, haemorrhage, varicose eczema (61), or ankle oedema.

Varicose veins may undoubtedly cause aching, and seem also to predispose to nocturnal cramps, but aching legs are very common in patients who do not have varicose veins. Patients are commonly referred for treatment of veins where symptoms are due to arthritis, arterial disease, musculoskeletal pain, and many other conditions. Alternative explanations should be searched for, as treating the veins will confer no benefit if they are not the cause of the symptoms. Aching felt broadly over the distribution of the varicosities, which is exacerbated by prolonged standing and relieved by putting the legs up, may well be due to the varicose veins, especially if valvular incompetence and reflux in the veins can be demonstrated (see facing page).

Ankle oedema may be due to varicose veins, but is more common when deep venous reflux is also present. Alternative causes should be excluded. Haemorrhage from varicose veins is remarkably uncommon, except in a small minority of patients in whom the varicosities appear to be eroding through the skin. Surgical treatment may be necessary to prevent further bleeding.

Brown staining of the skin in and around the ankle (due to haemosiderin deposition) is a benign phenomenon. Varicose veins may, however, give rise to a troublesome itchy eczema near the ankles, which may then spread to other parts of the body. Of most concern is the thickening, pigmentation, and hyperkeratosis (lipodermatosclerosis) which may develop in severe chronic venous insufficiency and predispose to ulceration.

Past medical history

A history suggestive of previous deep vein thrombosis, DVT, (pain with swelling of the leg) should be sought, although two-thirds of DVTs are believed to be asymptomatic and a negative response does not exclude the diagnosis. A previous DVT suggests that the deep venous system may be damaged but, more importantly, it is a major risk factor for a further DVT in a patient who may be considered for surgical treatment. Details of other past or concurrent medical conditions should similarly be obtained, as a basis for deciding whether or not to offer surgery. Varicose veins commonly run in families (sometimes even running true to one leg).

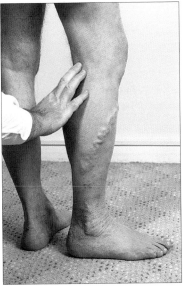

59 Severe varicose veins.

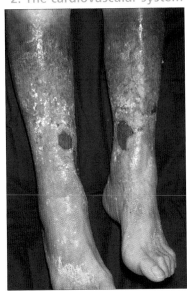

60 Ulceration caused by varicose veins.

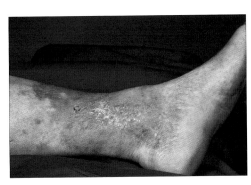

61 Varicose eczema.

Examination of the patient

General observation

The patient's general state of health should be noted. Advanced age, severe immobility, obesity, dyspnoea, and other debilitating conditions may all, to a greater or lesser extent, be contraindications to treatment or may affect choice of treatment.

Inspection of the legs

The extent and distribution of varicose veins is best observed with the patient standing. The distribution is an unreliable guide to the system which is affected, however. In particular, varicosities confined to the posteromedial aspect of the calf may fill either via the long or the short saphenous system. Varicose veins in the thigh are nonetheless likely to be associated with saphenofemoral incompetence and reflux in the long saphenous vein, while varicosities on the back of the calf suggest short saphenopopliteal reflux.

The condition of the skin should also be noted. Pigmentation alone is harmless, but the presence of eczema or lipodermatosclerosis (61) is important.

Detection and localization of reflux

Palpation With the patient standing, the upper ends of the long and short saphenous veins can often be palpated. (The knee should be slightly bent when examining the short saphenous vein.) A dilated and tense vein suggests the presence of reflux, and a varicose upper end of the long saphenous (saphena varix) is diagnostic. A slight cough impulse over the saphenofemoral junction is not abnormal, but a strong impulse – especially if associated with a thrill – is also indicative of incompetence.

3 The respiratory system

Respiratory diseases often lead to hospital admission and patients with chronic obstructive airways disease may require repeated admissions for infective exacerbations. Carcinoma of the bronchus is the most common cause of cancer death in men, and its prevalence in women has increased in recent years. In the UK, the incidence of pulmonary tuberculosis has increased since 1987, with a similar trend being observed in other Western countries. There is a greater awareness of asthma by the general public, surveys indicating an increasing prevalence in both adults and children. Public concern about industrial pollution has led to industry adopting greater safeguards but, nevertheless, occupational lung disease remains an important clinical problem. Smoking remains the single most important cause of respiratory disease despite greater awareness of the dangers of cigarette smoking and health warnings placed on advertisements and cigarette packets. For instance, there has been only a small decline in the total numbers of smokers in the UK during the past years.

Examination of the nose has been included in this section, as common illnesses affecting the respiratory tract often present with 'upper respiratory tract', or 'coryzal', symptoms. This is the case with the common cold.

The nose

Applied anatomy and physiology

The nose comprises the external nose and the two nasal cavities (**62**). The external nose is given its pyramidal shape by the nasal septum, which articulates with the frontal bone. The nasal cavities form the first part of the respiratory passage and extend from the anterior nares or nostrils to the nasopharynx. The nares are lined with respiratory epithelium, with some olfactory epithelium. The cavities are separated by a midline septum, formed from septal cartilage.

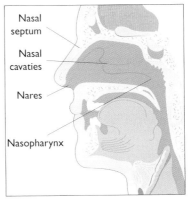

62 Anatomy of the nose.

The lateral wall of the nose has a large surface area due to the presence of three bony projections – the nasal conchae. The nose receives its nerve supply from the maxillary nerve in the anterior ethmoidal branch of the ophthalmic nerve; the upper part of the nasal cavity is supplied by the olfactory nerve. Lymphatic drainage is to the submandibular nodes and retropharyngeal nodes. The nose is associated with the paranasal air sinuses, the frontal, ethmoidal, sphenoidal, and maxillary sinuses.

Assessment and diagnosis

Taking the history

Patients present with symptoms of nasal obstruction, or of a change in his/her sense of smell. Any assessment of the patient begins by observation during history taking.

The presenting complaint

Nasal obstruction This is one of the most common nasal symptoms, most frequently resulting from the common cold. Patients present with a short history of nasal obstruction and discharge. Other causes of nasal obstruction include polyps, and allergic rhinitis.

Nasal discharge This may be watery, mucoid, mucopurulent, or bloodstained. It is important to ask for details. Sneezing is commonly associated with both nasal obstruction and nasal discharge.

Sense of smell Sense of smell is often reduced in inflammatory disorders of the nose; however both loss of, and alteration to, the sense of smell can also be caused by a cranial nerve lesion affecting the first cranial nerve.

Physical aspects Finally, it is important to ask about any deformity of the nose. Nasal symptoms can be caused by deviation of the nasal septum as a result of previous trauma. The nasal septum can also be affected by a Wegener's granulomatosus, syphilis, and leprosy.

Examination of the nose

Look for the shape of the nose in the presence of any deformity or scars. Check the nasal cavities with a nasal speculum. In a child, it is sufficient to look with a pen light. Inspection of the nasopharynx is possible, but only with the use of a post-nasal mirror.

The lungs

Applied anatomy and physiology

The respiratory tract includes the nose, nasopharynx, and larynx extending down into the alveoli to include the blood supply. An understanding of the arrangement of the lobes of the lungs is important for a clinical assessment, and this is illustrated in **63**. The right lung is divided into three lobes – upper, middle, and lower, while the left lung is divided into two lobes – the upper and lower, with the lingula (an incomplete left middle lobe) dividing the two.

Examination of the front of the chest is largely that of the upper lobes, whereas examination of the back is largely the lower lobes. It should be noted, however, that right middle lobe disease will only be detected by careful examination of the front of the chest and axillary area – signs of a right middle lobe pneumonia are often missed.

The muscular effort of inspiration overcomes the elastic resistance of the lungs and chest wall and the non-elastic resistance which is predominantly found in the airways. In normal subjects the large central airways contribute most resistance, with less from small airways due to the larger combined

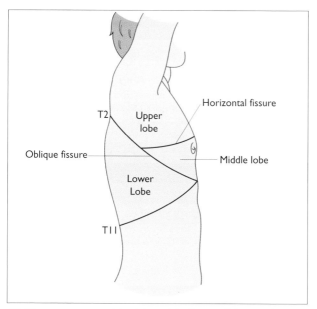

63 The arrangement of the lobes of the lung, and their surface markings.

cross-sectional area. In disease, resistance of either kind will greatly increase and call into action accessory muscles of inspiration (sternomastoid and scaleni) or expiration (abdominals). Examples of altered respiratory resistance are listed in **Table 16**. Gas exchange in the lungs will only be efficient if ventilation is distributed evenly to all parts of the lungs, and this is matched by uniform distribution of blood flow. Furthermore, this also requires effective diffusion of carbon dioxide and oxygen along the terminal airways and across the alveolar wall.

If the area available for gas exchange is reduced, or if the effective area is decreased by maldistribution of ventilation and perfusion, the overall ability of the lung to transfer gases will also diminish. Such a reduction may not be physiologically significant at rest, but may limit the amount of oxygen which can be taken up during exercise.

Table 16. Disorders causing an alteration in respiratory resistance

Elastic resistance – increased
- Pulmonary fibrosis
- Pulmonary oedema
- Kyphoscoliosis
- Ankylosing spondylitis

Elastic resistance – decreased
- Emphysema

Non-elastic resistance (airway resistance)
- Asthma
- Emphysema
- Chronic bronchitis

Assessment and diagnosis of respiratory disease

The assessment of a patient with respiratory disease follows the guidelines for general history taking. Some of the questions asked may overlap with those used for assessing the cardiovascular system.

Taking the history

The six cardinal symptoms of respiratory disease are cough, sputum, haemoptysis, chest pain, dyspnoea, and wheeze. These are all unpleasant symptoms which may make the patient tired or too distressed to answer questions easily. Ensure that the patient is sitting up and do not remove an oxygen mask, if the patient has one, while you are speaking to him/her; the patient will feel more comfortable this way. As for the cardiovascular system, remember to start your history with an open question.

The presenting complaint

Cough Cough is the forced expulsion of air through a closed glottis. The tracheobronchial tree is richly supplied with mucosal cough receptors, the fibres from which are carried in the vagus nerve. Irritation of these receptors anywhere from the pharynx to the periphery of the lung may initiate coughing. Cough may be caused by infection, inflammation, tumour, or foreign body – the full history will help you decide the cause. Cough may be the only symptom in asthma, so ask:

- 'Does your cough occur after exercise or at night?', as this may suggest cough due to bronchospasm.

Many smokers regard coughing as normal, so you should enquire about a change in its character, as this may be important:

- 'I understand that you have had a cough for many years. Tell me if it has changed recently'.

Patients can often localize a cough either above or below the larynx. A post-nasal drip from rhinitis is an example of the former, which may be associated with a chronically blocked nose. Laryngitis is usually associated with both a cough and a hoarse voice, whereas the appearance of a hoarse voice alone should raise the suspicion of a recurrent laryngeal nerve palsy due to carcinoma of the bronchus.

Try to separate these symptoms in your questioning. The cough in tracheitis is often dry and extremely painful behind the trachea, and is associated with pain on coughing. Cough is also associated with lobar pneumonia and lung collapse due to bronchial obstruction – the two conditions may be accompanied by pleurisy, making the cough distressingly painful over the lungs.

One of the most common causes of coughing is chronic bronchitis, which leads to a chronic or recurrent increase in the volume of mucus secretion that is expectorated. An accepted clinical definition for chronic bronchitis is 'a chronic, or recurrent cough, with sputum on most days for at least three months of the year for two consecutive years'. It is worth targeting your questions to establish whether this is the case:

- 'How long have you had this cough? Do you cough every day? Do you bring up sputum or phlegm – what colour is it?'

Ask the patient whether he/she has coughed up any blood (haemoptysis). Carcinoma of the bronchus is frequently associated with haemoptysis which may also be seen in pulmonary tuberculosis.

- 'Have you ever noticed blood in your phlegm?'

Frank haemoptysis is when pure blood is expectorated with sputum. It is essential to confirm that the blood is coming from the lungs and not the nose or mouth, or if it is being vomited. The volume and duration of haemoptysis must be noted.

Table 17. Different types of cough

Type of cough	Cause
Paroxysmal	Chronic bronchitis, asthma
Copious volume	Bronchiectasis
Painful	Pneumonia with pleurisy
'Bovine' (sounding like a cow)	Recurrent laryngeal palsy
Associated stridor	Whooping cough or partial laryngeal/tracheal obstruction

Bronchiectasis is characterized by a cough productive of copious sputum, which is often purulent and very offensive. Other less common causes of cough are from the inhalation of foreign bodies (the patient is generally unwell and pyrexial) and parenchymal lung disease (e.g. fibrosing alveolitis). Examples of different types of cough are shown in **Table 17**. The common causes of haemoptysis are shown in **Table 18**.

Sputum It is important to ask all patients with a cough whether they produce sputum or 'phlegm' – this is excessive bronchial secretion, and may be a manifestation of inflammation and infection. You should also ask how often they cough up sputum, and if it is difficult to bring up. You should question about the volume of sputum, its colour, its consistency, and its smell.

- 'How much phlegm do you cough up each day – would it fill an egg cup or a teacup?'
- 'What is it like – is it runny or thick?'
- 'What does it smell like?'

Table 18. Common causes of haemoptysis

- Bronchial carcinoma
- Pulmonary tuberculosis
- Pulmonary embolism and infarction
- Infection involving bronchiectasis
- Pulmonary oedema
- Anticoagulation
- Upper respiratory tract infection (acute bronchitis)
- No cause found

Characteristics of phlegm

- *Colour* – sputum is generally described as being either white or grey in colour, the latter particularly by cigarette smokers. In infection, the colour will often change to yellow (due to the presence of leukocytes) or green (as a result of enzymatic action by verdoperoxidase). Sticky and 'rusty' sputum is characteristic of lobar pneumonia, while pink, frothy sputum suggests pulmonary oedema.

- *Consistency* – highly viscous sputum with plugs is characteristic of asthma. Viscous sputum is also occasionally associated with viral respiratory infections.

- *Odour* – offensive sputum is seen in association with a lung abscess or bronchiectasis.

Chest pain (see also Chapter 2) The most common type of pain coming from the respiratory system is pleural pain due to the rich nerve supply of the parietal pleura (the lungs have no such nerve supply). The pain is described as localized and stabbing in nature, and is made worse by any manoeuvre which apposes the pleural surfaces, such as deep breathing, coughing, or sneezing. A similar pain is sometimes seen in association with a pneumothorax. Pain in the shoulder tip suggests irritation of the diaphragmatic pleura, whereas a dull, 'boring' pain may represent rib erosion by carcinoma of the bronchus. Pain localized to the anterior chest may be accompanied by tenderness on palpation of the costochondral junction as a result of costochondritis.

The questions to ask include:
- 'Does it hurt when you breathe?'
- 'What is the pain like?'
- 'Is it there all the time?'

Breathlessness Most types of lung disease will cause dyspnoea or difficulty in breathing. It is important to determine the degree of shortness of breath and the resulting functional disability (i.e. how much activity the individual can undertake). Patients will often complain of 'tightness' in the chest which may result either from angina or lung disease. You should ask the patient to distinguish whether he/she means pain associated with exercise or breathlessness, but remember that the latter may accompany angina.

Breathlessness may result from the following, either individually or as a combination:

- Altered ventilatory drive to the lungs.
- Impaired ventilation of the lungs.
- Altered gas exchange (or diffusion).
- Changes in perfusion of the lungs.

Examples of such causes are listed in **Table 19**. You should question a patient about the duration of the dyspnoea, and its variability. Acute dyspnoea may result from a pulmonary embolism, pneumothorax, or acute asthma, while progressive dyspnoea over a period of years suggests chronic airways limitation – particularly in the cigarette smoker. Questions about daily activities are helpful to determine more clearly how long the dyspnoea has been present –

Table 19. Causes of breathlessness

- *Alterations in the ventilatory drive:*
  Hyperventilation syndrome
  Obesity–hypoventilatory syndrome
  Hypothalamic lesions

- *Alterations in ventilatory capacity:*
  Neuromuscular disease
  Mechanical problems:
  - Kyphoscoliosis
  - Ankylosing spondylitis
  - Pleural effusion

- *Altered gas exchange (ventilation and/or diffusion):*
  Chronic bronchitis and emphysema
  Asthma
  Bronchiectasis
  Fibrosing alveolitis
  Pneumonia
  Pneumothorax
  Lung collapse
  Pulmonary oedema

- *Altered blood supply (perfusion):*
  Pulmonary embolism or lung infarction
  Anaemia

you should ask the patient how far he/she can walk on good days, and when he/she last visited shops if currently housebound. Remember always to gauge a patient's exercise capacity. In many instances a spouse or partner may give more reliable answers.

Variability of the dyspnoea:

- 'Does your breathlessness come and go?' – is highly suggestive of asthma, particularly if the patient can describe precipitating or aggravating factors.

Wheeze Most patients understand the term 'wheeze', which is a common complaint in patients with diffuse airways obstruction such as chronic bronchitis, emphysema, and asthma. Wheezing in patients with chronic bronchitis or patients with emphysema may result from further narrowing of the airways by an inter-current infection, whereas wheezing in asthmatics may be induced by exposure to an inhaled allergen. A unilateral wheeze should raise concerns about localized bronchial narrowing, either by a tumour or a foreign body.

Other important points from the history

You should ask the patient about his/her weight. Weight loss may be associated with carcinoma of the bronchus, pulmonary tuberculosis, and, on occasions, with chronic airflow limitation. The sleep apnoea syndrome, which is common in obese patients – and particularly those with a large neck circumference – may present with sleep disturbance and restlessness at night, loud snoring, and daytime somnolence. The patient may not complain of these factors, but they may come to light when questioning a spouse or partner or from their reporting.

- 'Does your wife complain that you snore? Has she ever noticed that you stop breathing for a period during the night?'

It is important to ask about this problem, as chronic nocturnal hypoxia can cause pulmonary hypertension and heart failure.

Past history

It is essential to take an accurate history of any previous chest complaints, injuries, or operations. A previous history of tuberculosis is important, and you should enquire about the length of treatment and/or operative intervention (such as thoracoplasty or phrenic nerve crush, which were commonly performed treatment for pulmonary TB before the introduction of streptomycin in 1947). A history of childhood asthma, pneumonia, or whooping cough are sometimes relevant to the later development of chest symptoms in an adult. Chest injuries and previous pneumonia may explain changes seen on a chest X-ray.

Personal and social history

Passive smoking (i.e. inhaling someone else's smoke at home or in the workplace) is now recognized as a risk for lung disease. Household pets are occasionally associated with chest symptoms, in particular asthma in allergic individuals. Progressive dyspnoea in a person who keeps birds (e.g. pigeons, budgerigars, parrots) may suggest allergic alveolitis, while pneumonia in someone who keeps a parrot or related species raises the possibility of psittacosis.

A detailed occupational history is essential – you should ask the patient whether his/her work provokes the symptoms, and whether these impair his/her work. Industrial exposure to noxious gases or particles may be a cause of lung disease – for example, pneumoconiosis in coal miners. You should also enquire about past employment – asbestosis or mesothelioma may not present until many years after exposure. Finally, a question about possible environmental exposure is helpful – remember that relatives of those who worked in contact with asbestos are also at risk.

Family and treatment history

There is a strong inherited component to asthma, and you should enquire about a history of atopy, asthma, or eczema in the family. Moreover, you should question, if relevant, about recent tuberculosis in the family. The treatment history should question about the past and present use of bronchodilator inhalers, and how useful they may or may not be. You should also enquire whether any drugs, such as aspirin, non-steroidal anti-inflammatory agents or ß-blockers, have precipitated an asthmatic attack or wheezing in the past. Remember also the possible dangers of steroid therapy in patients with a previous history of tuberculosis.

Examination of the patient

The patient with respiratory system disease may be short of breath, so it is important to keep this in mind, and not keep asking him/her to sit forwards and back. Examine everything you can from the front first, then ask the patient to sit forward and repeat the process from behind.

In addition, breathlessness makes people feel tired and anxious. Make sure to remember this – and be patient.

Social history

A detailed social history must be taken, which includes a smoking history. You should substantiate whether the non-smoker has previously smoked and, if so, when s/he gave up – many patients 'give up' on admission to hospital. Examples of the questions to ask include:

- 'Do you smoke?'
- 'When did you start?'
- 'How many cigarettes do you smoke in an average day?'(NB: pack/years)
- 'When did you give up?'
- 'How many were you smoking when you gave up?'

Checklist for respiratory history taking

- General approach, introduce yourself establish rapport, eye contact.

- Assess the present complaint and its history (duration of breathlessness, exercise tolerance). Don't forget to ask about cigarette smoking.

- Ask about past medical history, particularly in relation to childhood chest complaints, and previous hospital attendance.

- Ask about alcohol intake/treatment and medication use.

- Ask about social history, e.g. how many stairs, heating in the home, pets, industrial exposure. You may include the smoking history here.

- Ask about family history – does anyone have asthma or other chronic respiratory illness?

- Systematic enquiry.

LISTEN TO THE ANSWERS!

General observations

Observe the general shape of the chest, looking for asymmetry and deformities such as depressed sternum, pigeon chest, or kyphoscoliosis (a hunch back). Observe the chest during both normal and deep breathing, and check that the two sides move equally. Diminished movement on one side suggests a lesion on that side. Note if the thoracic cage expands normally, or if it is fixed and the respiratory movements are predominantly diaphragmatic – observe the respiratory rate. A normal rate is approximately 12 cycles per minute.

As with the cardiovascular system, it is customary to begin with inspection of the hands, with the patient lying in bed with the chest at a 45° angle. Look for finger clubbing (**14**), which is described as an increase in the curvature of the nails in both directions, with loss of the nail angle. This is caused by an increase in the soft tissues of the nail bed and finger tip. It is sometimes subtle and difficult to detect. In these cases, it is worthwhile looking for the diamond sign shown in **64**. In a normal individual, when the finger nails are opposed, a small, diamond-shaped gap can been seen between the base of the nails. In clubbing, this gap is not visible due to loss of the angle of the nail. There are long lists available of causes of clubbing which will not be duplicated here, but remember the more common intrapulmonary ones: bronchial carcinoma, chronic chest sepsis, fibrosing alveolitis. Also look for the signs of CO_2 retention – these are: a bounding pulse, and warm hands with dilated peripheral veins. Look for a flapping tremor by asking the patient to hold his/her hands out – a flapping tremor is an irregular twitching movement of the hands. The patient with a high level of CO_2 may also be peripherally cyanosed.

Following your examination of the patient's hands, make sure to look at the face. Is the patient centrally cyanosed, i.e. is there cyanosis of the mouth and tongue? Is s/he breathing out through pursed lips? This is a technique developed by people with chronic airflow limitation to keep their airways open to the end of the respiratory cycle, and increase their oxygenation. Look at the patient's neck to assess whether he/she is using the accessory muscles of respiration.

When the work required to achieve normal ventilation is increased, there will be a larger than normal fall in intrathoracic pressure on inspiration, and this will lead to the use of accessory muscles. Scalenus anterior is the first accessory muscle to be brought into use, followed by the sternomastoids – the latter can be seen contracting. When there is a considerable increase in the respiratory work, there will be a large fall of pressure within the chest on inspiration, and recession or indrawing of the intercostal muscles is then easily visible.

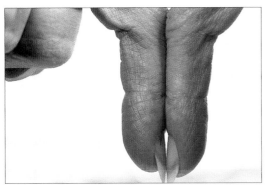

64 The diamond sign: in normal individuals, a diamond shape can be seen between the nail folds. This disappears if the patient's fingers are clubbed.

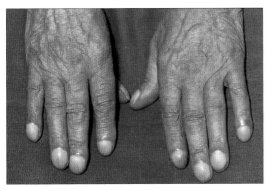

65 Clubbing and peripheral cyanosis in fibrosing alveolitis.

An increase in respiratory work may result either from an increase in airways resistance or an increase in lung stiffness (see **Table 16**, page 82). The pattern of abnormal intrathoracic pressure changes will vary according to the cause of increased work, and this may be discernible at the bedside. When there is increased airways resistance (e.g. asthma), expiration is impeded and the respiratory phase of breathing is prolonged. This can be demonstrated by asking a patient to breath out as fast as he/she can. By contrast, when there is an increase in lung stiffness (e.g. fibrosing alveolitis, **65**), expiration is aided by elastic recoil and the chest/lungs may often be seen to deflate unusually fast.

Check to see whether the costal margins expand laterally during a deep inspiration. The ribs normally move upward and outward when the chest inflates (like a bucket handle). Failure to expand, or actual indrawing of the lowest ribs, suggests a flattened diaphragm and a lung volume larger than normal.

You will have already noted whether the jugular venous pressure (JVP) is raised when examining the cardiovascular system (CVS). The patient with severe respiratory disease may have associated right heart failure with elevated JVP and swollen ankles.

Finally, look for enlarged lymph nodes in the anterior and posterior triangles of the neck (66), as lymphatic drainage from the lungs is first to the hilum, then up the paratracheal chain to the supraclavicular and cervical nodes. Chest wall lymphatics drain into the axillae and may produce lymphadenopathy: a carcinoma of the bronchus may metastasize here. These lymph nodes are most easily examined from behind by placing your fingertips first in the supraclavicular fossae, and then working up the root of the neck on either side of the sternomastoid muscle to the jugulodigastric node at the angle of the jaw, and then the submandibular nodes.

To examine the axillary nodes, support the patient's arm a little away from the chest wall (use your left hand to examine the right axilla, and right hand to examine the left axilla). Palpate anteriorly, posteriorly, medially, laterally, and in the apex of the axilla (67). (A more detailed technique is discussed in Chapter 7.) Abnormal lymph nodes are larger than you expect (lymphadenopathy). They may be enlarged asymmetrically, and may feel hard and fixed in the case of metastases.

Examination of the chest itself follows the sequence inspection, palpation, percussion, auscultation.

Inspection of the chest

You should next inspect the patient's chest. This is best done with the patient sitting relaxed and bare-chested in front of you. Respiratory disease often results in alteration of the normal chest shape. You should compare the two sides of the chest from the front and back to look for any obvious asymmetry (68). Also inspect the patient from the side, to assess the antero-posterior diameter, and whether s/he has a kyphosis. This is an increased antero-posterior curvature of the spine which will increase the diameter of the chest from front to back. There is a wide variation in chest shape among normal individuals, and the only way to become familiar with the normal range is to examine a large number of patients. The chest wall may be held in hyperinflation – the barrel chest – as a result of chronic airflow limitation. Apical fibrosis and scarring may result in flattening of the chest at one or both apices.

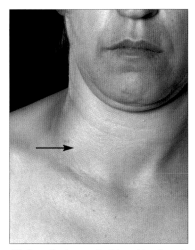

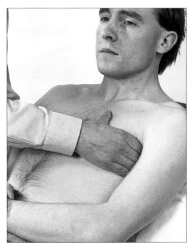

66 Lymphadenopathy. Note blurring of the sternomastoid border on the right (arrow).

67 Palpation of axillary lymphadenopathy.

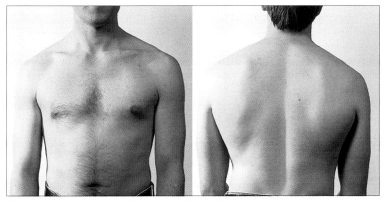

68 Inspect the chest from the front and from the back.

It is also important to look again at the movement of the chest wall. To do this, ask the patient to take a few deep breaths in and out. The ribs should move upwards and outwards with inspiration, and this movement should be symmetrical (**69**). In chronic airflow limitation, there is little movement as the ribs are already fixed in the expanded position, while in asymmetrical scarring after tuberculosis, movement is greater on one side than another. As the patient breathes, listen for stridor, a harsh noise made by respiratory obstruction in the upper respiratory tract. Make sure you check for any scars on the chest indicative of previous surgery or trauma.

The rest of the examination of the chest needs to be performed on the front and back. It is sensible to complete the examination of the front *before* asking the patient to sit forwards so as not to tire him/her. This will include chest expansion, percussion, and auscultation.

Palpation and assessment of chest expansion Look at the position of the trachea between the heads of the two sternomastoid muscles, and observe for a tug or downwards pulling movement of the skin over the trachea, which you may see in respiratory distress. Next, gently palpate the trachea: using your right hand, place the tips of your index and middle finger to either side of the trachea, and gently feel in the sulcus on either side to gain an impression of the direction the trachea is running, and whether it is deviated to the right or left. Deviation may be caused by masses in the neck, but can also be due to mediastinal shift. If this is suspected, it can be confirmed by palpating the apex beat, to see whether this is also deviated to the right or left.

To examine chest expansion, place your flat hands around the patient's chest, just below the nipple line (or the breasts in women), with your thumbs stretched out towards the midline and slightly off the skin, and ask the patient to breathe in deeply. Watch your thumbs move apart, and check that they move an equal amount. This procedure should be repeated at the back of the chest.

Percussion In percussion and auscultation of the chest, the aim is to compare one side with the other. It is essential to percuss or auscultate systematically to ensure you do not miss any areas. An example of such a system is illustrated in **70** and **71**.

To percuss, the non-dominant hand should be placed flat against the chest wall, and the back of the middle finger is tapped lightly by the middle finger of the other hand. It is important to tap with your finger tip perpendicular to the middle finger (keep this nail short, otherwise it digs into your other finger). Keep your wrist relaxed, and ensure that most of the movement comes from here, not your elbow.

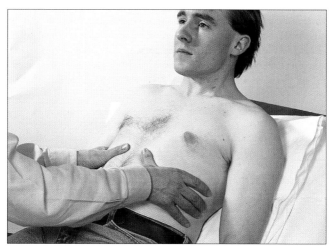

69 Palpation of chest expansion.

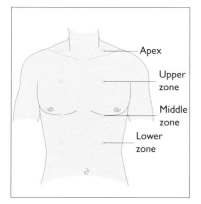

70 Areas for chest examination (anterior).

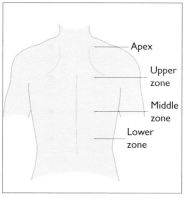

71 Areas for chest examination (posterior).

It is important to start at the apices, by percussing over the clavicles. This can be done by percussing directly onto the bone. Next, compare one side with the other side in the upper, middle, and lower zones. It is important to percuss in the axilla as well as the front and back of the chest; abnormalities of the right middle lobe or lingula may only be apparent here. The percussion note is a measure of the resonance of the chest wall. As the lungs are normally filled with air (hollow), the percussion note is normally resonant. If the intrathoracic space is filled by collapsed or consolidated lung, the percussion note will be dull (as solid material conducts sound less well than air – 72). If the space is filled with fluid – as in a pleural effusion – the percussion note will be stony dull (73), as fluid conducts vibration very poorly. If the intrathoracic cavity is filled by air, as in a pneumothorax, the percussion note will be hyper-resonant (74). An illustration of the relationship of some clinical conditions to their percussion notes is shown in **Table 20**.

Table 20. Conditions affecting conduction of sound through the chest wall

Problem	Chest wall movement	Trachea position	Percussion note	Tactile vocal fremitus	Breath sounds
Consolidation:	Normal	Central	Dull	↑	↑ + Bronchial breathing
Collapse (large airways):	Reduced	Deviated towards lesion	Dull	↓	↓↓↓ or absent
Collapse (small airways):	Normal	Central or →	Normal or ↓	Normal (but vesicular)	Normal
Pleural effusion:	Reduced	Deviated away from the lesion	Dull	↓	↓↓↓ May be bronchial above the fluid + aegophony
Pneumothorax (large):	Reduced	Central or deviated away from the scale of the lesion	Normal	Absent	Absent – sounds conducted from the other side

↑ = increased
↓ = decreased
→ = towards

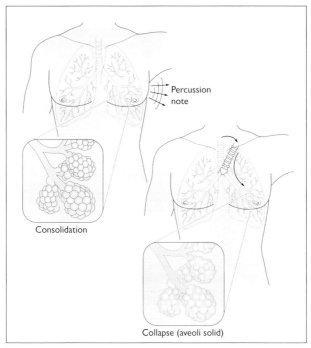

Consolidation

Collapse (aveoli solid)

72 In consolidation, the percussion note is 'dull'.

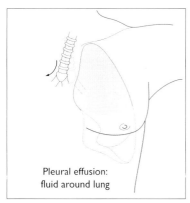

Pleural effusion:
fluid around lung

73 In a pleural effusion, the percussion note is 'stony dull'.

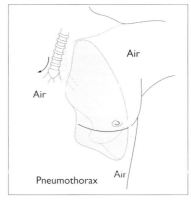

Pneumothorax

74 In pneumothorax, the percussion note is increased.

Auscultation As with percussion, in auscultation it is important to listen over an area on one side, and then compare this directly with the other side (**75**). The diaphragm of the stethoscope should be used for this. Ask the patient to breathe in, and then to breathe right out through an open mouth. Listen over the apices of both lungs first, then over the upper, middle and lower zones, followed by the axillae. Repeat the auscultation when examining the patient's chest. While listening, it is important to concentrate on the breath sounds themselves, and to listen for added sounds. Normal breath sounds are termed 'vesicular' in nature.

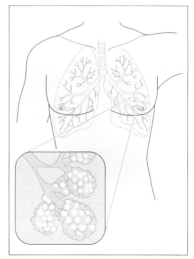

75 The percussion note is dull, with reduced sounds, as the air passages are occluded in collapse.

Sounds These are produced by the movement of air in and out of normal lung tissue and airways. They are heard over all normal lung tissue, with no clear pause between inspiration and expiration, and come from the region immediately below the stethoscope. Bronchial sounds are much more harsh, with a clear pause between inspiration and expiration, and a prolonged expiratory phase. They are dominated by the glottic hiss, which is transmitted from the larynx, and can be heard normally over the trachea and large airways. In health, they are not heard elsewhere, except in expiration. If the lung tissue becomes solid due to consolidation, there is increased conduction of this bronchial-quality sound to the chest wall, with a reduction in the normal vesicular breathing as air entry is reduced or absent. This is called bronchial breathing, and is best heard over the area affected by the consolidation. In consolidation, the alveoli are full of inflammatory exudate but the air passages remain open; this differentiates consolidation from collapse, where the air passages are occluded (see **Table 20**, page 96) and bronchial breathing is not heard.

Vocal resonance Different frequencies of voice sounds are transmitted to the chest wall, and these frequencies are increased, decreased, or altered in disease states (see **Table 20**, page 96). This can be assessed clinically by asking the patient to say 'ninety-nine' or 'one, one, one', while listening to the chest.

The spoken voice sounds hollow through a stethoscope placed over normal lung, as low-pitched sounds are transmitted better than high-pitched sounds.

Altered vocal resonance is best heard over areas of consolidation, and is best described as an increase of the clarity of the words heard (with an almost booming nature) through the chest wall. This sign is called bronchophony, and is due to the increased sound-conducting properties of solid tissue over air. If vocal resonance is present, it may be easier to hear as 'whispering pectoriloquy'. The whispered voice is conducted very clearly, as it consists largely of high-frequency noises – almost like being in a whispering gallery.

When there is a pleural effusion, the spoken voice heard through the stethoscope is high-pitched, with a nasal quality known as aegophony: this occurs because the improved transmission of high frequencies is accompanied by impaired transmission of the lower frequencies. ('Aegophony' means goat-voice, because of its bleating quality.)

Tactile vocal fremitus Vibration of the chest wall is also assessed by palpation. This can be done at this stage, although is sometimes easier to put into context at the end of the examination of the chest. This test for the transmission of low-frequency vibrations is closely related to auscultation findings, as an increase in tactile vocal fremitus (vibration) is associated with an increase in sound conduction through the chest wall. Place the flat of your hand on the patient's chest, and ask the patient to say 'ninety-nine'. Compare one side with the other over the front and back of the chest in the areas illustrated in **69** and **70**. The degree of vibration over each lung should be compared.

Added sounds Crackles and wheezes are the most common added sounds you are likely to encounter. Crackles are produced by air bubbles bursting through fluid in the alveoli. They are described as fine or coarse. The noise of fine crackles can be reproduced by rolling your hair between your finger and thumb just in front of your ear. These noises are usually heard at the end of inspiration. Fine crackles are heard in pulmonary oedema, and in early bronchopneumonias where they tend to be basal, and pulmonary fibrosis, where they may be more widespread.

Coarse crackles have a harsh, clicking sound, and are heard in infection or bronchiectasis.

Caring for the patient with respiratory system disease

- Appreciate their anxiety.
- Bed rest in a sitting position.
- Oxygen always available. Only 24% unless otherwise requested.
- Monitor peak expiratory flow rate (PEFR).
- Check respiratory rate regularly.
- Cardiac monitoring may be necessary.
- Weigh the patient daily – (in cases with coexistent heart failure).

A few basal crackles may be heard in the normal upright subject breathing quietly, and this probably results from airways closing in the dependent lung during shallow breathing – this is an effect of gravity. Characteristically, these crackles clear on coughing.

Pleural rub A pleural rub is a creaking sound, caused by the inflamed pleural surfaces rubbing against each other. Characteristically it sounds like creaking leather, and is usually located over an area of pleuritic pain. It is heard in both inspiration and expiration and can be confused with the noise made when listening to the chest through clothing – hence, always examine the bare chest.

Illustrated physical signs

Peripheral cyanosis with dilated veins is a feature of the CO_2 retention characteristic of chronic obstructive pulmonary disease (COPD) (76). A **kyphoscoliosis** (77) often predisposes a patient to respiratory disease. **Tuberculosis** at X-ray (78). A flattened upper chest is caused by fibrosis from previous **apical TB** (79); this patient also has angulation due to spinal involvement. **Bronchial carcinoma** (80). In a patient with **lobar pneumonia**, there is often coexistent oral herpes simplex infection (81, 82). In a **collapsed lung** (pneumothorax) no lung markings can be seen on the X-ray (83).

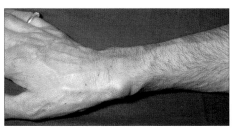

76 Peripheral cyanosis with dilated peripheral veins found in CO_2 retention.

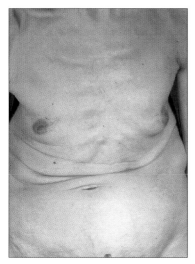

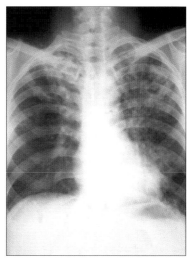

77 Kyphoscoliosis predisposes to respiratory disease.

78 Tuberculosis. Cavitation is seen in the upper lobes.

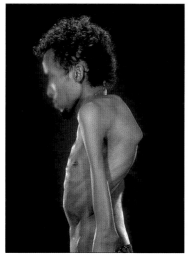

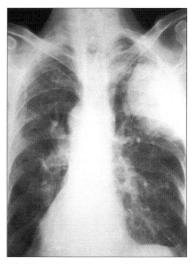

79 Apical tuberculosis. A flattened apex due to previous tuberculosis, with angulation due to spinal involvement.

80 Bronchial carcinoma. A large opacity is shown in the left upper zone.

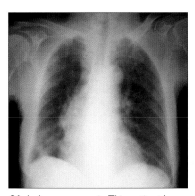

81 Lobar pneumonia. This patient has right-sided consolidation.

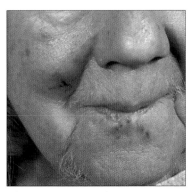

82 Herpes simplex infection is common in patients with lobar pneumonia.

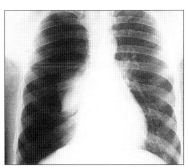

83 Right-sided pneumothorax with complete absence of lung markings.

Therapeutic and interventional skills

Peak expiratory flow rate (PEFR) measurement

You will need either a Wright's peak flow meter, or a smaller portable version. Ensure that you use a clean disposable mouth-piece for each patient. Ask the patient to take in a large breath through the mouth, then seal the lips around the tube and breathe out as quickly and forcefully as possible into the meter (as if blowing out

Findings in a normal respiratory system examination

- Observation – chest wall and respiratory movements are equal and symmetrical.
- Chest expansion, equal and symmetrical.
- Trachea, central.
- Percussion note resonant.
- Auscultation – breath sounds vesicular, no added sounds.
- Tactile vocal fremitus present and equal on both sides.

Arterial blood gas estimation

Arterial blood gases are used in the assessment of breathlessness. The results obtained provide vital clues to the underlying cause and the severity of the condition.

● Note the inspired O_2 concentration.

● Warn the patient that the procedure may be painful – and ask them to keep as still as possible. Outline the procedure to the patient, and make sure you have their verbal consent.

● If doing a radial puncture, ensure that the ulnar artery is palpable in that wrist and that it is able to perfuse the hand. You can use a simple manoeuvre to demonstrate this.

● Obstruct the radial artery by pressure from your fingertips. Ask the patient to close his/her fist tightly to expel remaining blood, keeping pressure on the radial artery. Then ask them to open the hand again. Flushing of the palm shows that ulnar artery perfusion is adequate.

● Open the blood gas syringe, which is pre-heparinized, and make sure that the heparin has coated the inside of the syringe by withdrawing and replacing the plunger. Expel the excess and attach the needle.

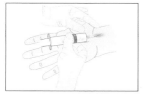

84 Blood gas sampling from the radial artery.

● Wearing sterile gloves, palpate the radial artery along its length, getting a feel for its direction. To sample arterial blood, insert the needle with the dominant hand, palpating the artery with the index and middle finger along its length (**84**). Advance the needle until arterial pressure fills the needle. Withdraw and apply pressure to the puncture site for 3 minutes with cotton wool. Seal the syringe with the bung, and take it in ice to the blood gas analysis machine.

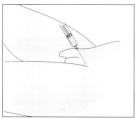

85 Femoral artery puncture.

● For a femoral puncture, remember that the nerve runs laterally to the artery, so err on the medial side. Clean the area thoroughly as it is near the groin. Use a 21-gauge needle, inserting it at 90° to the skin, using the dominant hand, and aim towards the pulsation, between the index and middle finger until the arterial pressure pushes blood into the syringe. Then proceed as for a radial puncture (**85**).

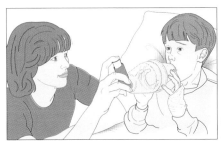

86 Spacer device being used in conjunction with an inhaler.

birthday cake candles). The patient must repeat this three times. This shifts the arrow in the gauge, and the highest recorded value is noted. It is often appropriate to do this before and after treatment with an inhaled bronchodilator, e.g. salbutamol. The normal PEFR is related to the patient's height – a normal value for a 1.83 m (6 ft) male is around 500–600 L/min.

Inhaler use

If a bronchodilator and steroid inhaler are to be used, the bronchodilator must be used first, in order to open the bronchioles and thus to maximize the delivery of the steroid. It is helpful to explain the procedure to the patient first, then instruct him/her step by step while they follow your instructions:

- Shake the inhaler vigorously; ask the patient to breathe in, then right out.
- Put the inhaler into his/her mouth and ask them to inhale deeply.
- At the beginning of the inspiration, tell them to press the plunger of the inhaler. This administers the active ingredient in a spray form, which is carried into the lungs with inspiration.
- Tell the patient to hold his/her breath for 10 seconds and then breathe out.
- Repeat after a pause if two puffs are required.

If the patient is unable to use an inhaler, a spacer device is available (**86**). This allows dispersal of the drug into a much larger volume of air. The inhaler is attached at one end, and the patient breathes in and out through the other. A one-way valve ensures delivery of the drug while the patient is breathing in. The other alternative is a rotahaler. With this technique, the patient breathes in and the drug delivery system is triggered by the rate of flow of inspired air.

Key laboratory tests

Arterial blood gas interpretation The arterial blood gas measurements indicate the oxygenation and degree of acidosis or alkalosis of the arterial blood.

Respiratory acidosis is caused by hypoventilation. The pH is low, $PaCO_2$ is high, and the plasma bicarbonate normal or raised. This may be compensated

Arterial blood gas measurement

Values vary from laboratory to laboratory, but a general range of normal values of arterial blood are:

PaO_2	12–13.5 kPa (85–95 mmHg)
$PaCO_2$	4.5–6.0 kPa (35–45 mmHg)
pH	7.35–7.45
Plasma bicarbonate (HCO_3)	20–30 mmol/L
Standard base excess (SBE)	± 2 mmol/L
% O_2 Saturation	95–100%

for if it is long-standing, giving a normal pH and a raised bicarbonate.

Respiratory alkalosis is caused by hyperventilation. The pH is high, $PaCO_2$ is low, and the plasma bicarbonate is normal or low.

The following illustrations depict the key features of common respiratory conditions: emphysema (**87**), primary carcinoma of the bronchus (**88**), asthma (**89**), pulmonary fibrosis (**90**), chronic obstructive pulmonary disease (**91**), and pulmonary tuberculosis (**92**).

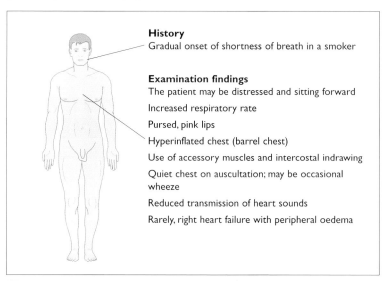

History
Gradual onset of shortness of breath in a smoker

Examination findings
The patient may be distressed and sitting forward

Increased respiratory rate

Pursed, pink lips

Hyperinflated chest (barrel chest)

Use of accessory muscles and intercostal indrawing

Quiet chest on auscultation; may be occasional wheeze

Reduced transmission of heart sounds

Rarely, right heart failure with peripheral oedema

87 Emphysema.

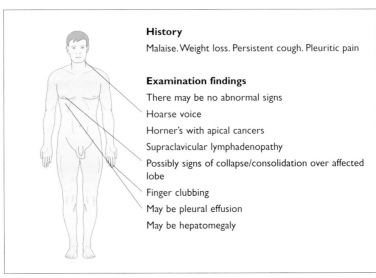

History

Malaise. Weight loss. Persistent cough. Pleuritic pain

Examination findings

There may be no abnormal signs

Hoarse voice

Horner's with apical cancers

Supraclavicular lymphadenopathy

Possibly signs of collapse/consolidation over affected lobe

Finger clubbing

May be pleural effusion

May be hepatomegaly

88 Primary carcinoma of the bronchus.

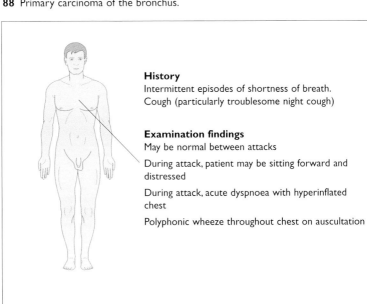

History

Intermittent episodes of shortness of breath. Cough (particularly troublesome night cough)

Examination findings

May be normal between attacks

During attack, patient may be sitting forward and distressed

During attack, acute dyspnoea with hyperinflated chest

Polyphonic wheeze throughout chest on auscultation

89 Asthma.

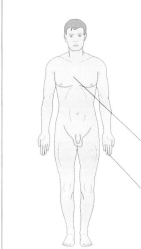

History
Progressive shortness of breath. There may be a past history of industrial exposure or associated connective tissue disease

Examination findings
There are widespread 'showers' of fine crackles that do not clear on coughing

The patient is breathless at rest

There may be finger clubbing

The patient may be cyanosed

90 Pulmonary fibrosis.

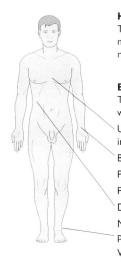

History
There is a history of productive cough for at least two months in any two consecutive years. The patient has repeated chest infections

Examination findings
The patient may be distressed and sitting forward, with increased respiratory rate. Barrel chest, blue lips

Using accessory muscles of respiration with intercostal indrawing

Bounding pulse and coarse tremor of fingers

Prolonged expiratory phase and expiratory wheezes

Possibly coarse crepitations

Downward displacement of liver

May be associated signs of right heart failure and peripheral oedema. Reduced heart sound transmissions

With severe CO_2 retention, mental confusion, drowsiness, coma, and papilloedema

91 Chronic obstructive pulmonary disease (COPD).

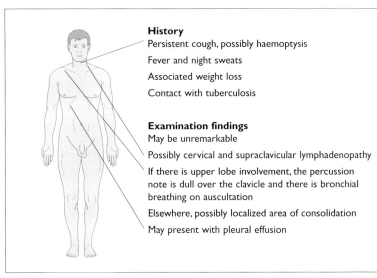

History
Persistent cough, possibly haemoptysis

Fever and night sweats

Associated weight loss

Contact with tuberculosis

Examination findings
May be unremarkable

Possibly cervical and supraclavicular lymphadenopathy

If there is upper lobe involvement, the percussion note is dull over the clavicle and there is bronchial breathing on auscultation

Elsewhere, possibly localized area of consolidation

May present with pleural effusion

92 Pulmonary tuberculosis.

4 The gastrointestinal system

Gastrointestinal disease is a common, and often asymptomatic cause of illness. A large number of patients have gastrointestinal symptoms but without organic disease. Differentiating between these two groups takes considerable clinical skill. It is important to reassure the patient with non-organic disease but, at the same time be certain that serious pathology is not being overlooked.

Applied anatomy and physiology of the gut

The basic anatomy of the gut is shown in **93**. The gastrointestinal tract is responsible for the ingestion of food, the absorption of nutrients from food, and the excretion of unabsorbed waste products. This process is controlled by the autonomic nervous system, together with hormones including gastrin, secretin, and cholecystokinin. The parasympathetic nervous system controls the contraction of smooth muscle and the secretion of digestive hormones. These are secreted in response to stretching of the gut, and to the presence of food in the upper gastrointestinal tract.

The **musculature** of the alimentary tract is composed of smooth muscle from the mid oesophagus to the external anal sphincter. Smooth muscle has an innate tone which permits sustained and sometimes powerful contraction over long periods of time. On the other hand, the muscle may respond to more gradual stretching by a decrease in tension and an increase in length. Smooth muscle activity is influenced both by neural and humoral components. The sympathetic nervous system has very little influence, while the parasympathetic system has a profound influence. Humoral influences on smooth muscle include those of neurohumoral

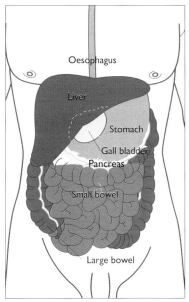

93 The basic anatomy of the gut.

transmitters (e.g. 5-hydroxytrytamine, prostaglandins), gastrointestinal hormones (e.g. glucagon), and drugs.

Gastric peristalsis occurs at a constant rate of three to four waves per minute. The pylorus, in contrast to the oesophageal sphincter, is not normally in a state of contraction, but at the end of each peristaltic wave it contracts together with the terminal antrum. Gastric emptying is proportional to the volume in the stomach, with about 1–3% of the gastric contents being emptied each minute. The rate of emptying is delayed by the presence of fat in the duodenum, a low pH, or hypertonic solution. This ensures that the duodenum is not overwhelmed by excessive amounts of hypertonic fluid, and that the intestinal contents are isotonic when they enter the jejunum. The body of the stomach secretes a juice whose main constituents are hydrochloric acid, pepsin, and intrinsic factor. Gastric secretion is secreted in three phases – cephalic (neural), gastric (hormonal), and intestinal (hormonal).

The most common movement of the **small intestine** are non-propulsive segmenting contractions whose main function is the mixing of intestinal contents. Peristaltic waves propel food along the lumen. The rate of passage through the duodenum is rapid, while the rate of transit in the ileum may be slow. The ileocaecal valve may further delay passage of the contents in the ileum, facilitating absorption of water and some nutrients. The exocrine pancreas secretes an aqueous juice with a high bicarbonate concentration and enzymic fluid containing the major proteolytic enzymes of digestion (trypsin, chymotrypsin, carboxypeptidase), amylase, and lipase. This secretion is controlled both by neural and hormonal mechanisms (secretin and cholecystokinin).

In the **large bowel,** most contractions are non-propulsive and serve to delay rather than promote transit. This accounts for the paradox that in diarrhoea, intraluminal pressure records show decreased activity and in constipation increased activity. After reception of food residues, the caecum exhibits mixing activity and then slowly contracts so that over six to ten hours food residues reach the transverse colon. One to three times each day, mass movements occur and propel the contents into the descending and sigmoid colon. Continence is maintained by two sphincters: the internal sphincter reflects the activity of the circular muscle of the intestine. Normally it is in tonic contraction. The external sphincter also shows continuous resting activity. Both the external and puborectalis muscle are inhibited on defaecation and micturition.

Although no glandular secretion occurs in the small and large intestines, there is a rapid exchange of water and electrolytes across parts of the **mucosa.** Water moves in response to osmotic gradients, a hypertonic solution being rapidly diluted by movement of water from blood to lumen and a hypotonic solution rapidly concentrated by absorption of water. Sodium is actively absorbed in both the small and large intestine, while potassium is absorbed by the small intestine but is secreted by the large intestine. Under normal circumstances, albumin leaks into the gut lumen in various secretions such as saliva, gastric juice, succus entericus, and bile. The exuded albumin is digested and the nitrogen subsequently absorbed as amino acids. This intestinal loss accounts for approximately 10% of the total albumin catabolism in the normal subject.

Assessment and diagnosis

Taking the history

A clear history of gastrointestinal symptoms is important, because it will often discriminate between organic and non-organic (functional) disease. Patients are often vague about symptoms, and may be embarrassed when discussing their bowel habit with the doctor. It is important for the practitioner to present as a sympathetic and caring individual, and it may be helpful to reassure the patient of the confidentiality of the consultation. It is also important to be very clear what the patient means by his/her symptoms. This is done using a combination of open questions to encourage the patient to describe symptoms in his/her own words, but with considerable reiteration and checking by the doctor, to make sure that the message is understood. The direction of the interview may also have to be guided, as patients may try to avoid embarrassing or intimate discussions. This can be done using closed and focused questions.

The presenting complaint

Any of the symptoms listed in **Table 21** may need to be explored with the patient.

Dysphagia The patient may complain that food sticks in their throat, or lower down on swallowing. You should establish where the food sticks, whether it is a consistent site, and whether it is more obvious with solids or liquids. Ask the patient to point to the area where he/she finds the food sticks:

- 'Tell me about the sensation you have of food sticking in your throat'.
- 'Where does it seem to stick?'
- 'Is it worse with drinks or solid food?'

Heartburn The patient complains of a burning sensation which occurs in the chest and may extend up into the throat. It is often positional, worse on lying down, and therefore also worse at night. It can be exacerbated by bending over, for example when doing up shoe laces. It is important to ensure that it is not

Table 21. Symptoms of gastrointestinal disease

- *Dysphagia* — Difficulty in swallowing
- *Heartburn* — Retrosternal burning sensation
- *Indigestion, dyspepsia* — Both of these are commonly used, but non-specific terms
- *Wind* — Describes flatulence, belching, or the passing of flatus
- *Nausea* — A feeling of impending vomiting
- *Retching* — Involuntary spasms with a desire to vomit
- *Vomiting* — Propulsive regurgitation of stomach contents
- *Diarrhoea* — Passing increased amounts of loose stool
- *Constipation* — Difficult passage of hard stool
- *Pain* — See text
- *Anorexia* — Loss of appetite
- *Colic* — Abdominal pain that waxes and wanes
- *Melaena* — Black stool (altered blood)
- *Tenesmus* — A painful urge to defaecate

related to exercise, as the symptoms of angina and heartburn can be difficult to differentiate:
- 'Describe the burning sensation. Where is it?'
- 'Does it go anywhere else? Is it related to food intake?'

Indigestion and dyspepsia These are vague terms, with a wide interpretation by patients. If the patient uses such terms it is important to establish exactly what he/she means, by closer questioning:
- 'Describe your indigestion to me. What is it like? When does it come on?'

Wind This term is usually used to describe belching or the passing of flatus. It can also be used to describe colicky (intermittent, but intense) abdominal pain. If the patient complains of wind, ask whether it tends to be passed downwards or upwards, and whether it relieves pain or other symptoms:
- 'Do you feel better after burping or passing wind?'

Nausea, retching, and vomiting These symptoms tend to occur together, but not always. It is important to inquire about the frequency of the symptoms, and whether they are related to pain. If vomiting is related to pain, does it bring relief? Ask about the approximate amount of vomitus and relate it to common things such as a tea cup, bowl or bucket. What colour is it, and does it have any traces of blood in it? Altered blood from the stomach is dark brown in appearance, and is called 'coffee grounds':

- 'Does the vomit taste sour, and does it contain foods? If so, how long ago were they eaten?'

Vomit containing undigested food suggests a possible delay in gastric emptying which may accompany pyloric stenosis.

Diarrhoea Establish the normal bowel habit, then ask about the change. Ask how many times the patient goes to the toilet to open his/her bowels, and compare this with his/her normal habit. Also ask about the volume and consistency of the stool:

- 'Is it formed, unformed or watery?'
- 'Does it smell, or float, and is it difficult to flush away?'
- 'Is there blood and/or mucus associated with the stool – if so, is it mixed in or on top of the stool?'
- 'Is there pain on defaecation, or before, and is it relieved by defaecation?'

Blood mixed in the stool suggests a possible neoplasm or chronic inflammatory bowel disease – blood on the lavatory paper is more suggestive of haemorrhoids. Both require further investigation.

Constipation Patients occasionally misunderstand the term constipation, so it is important to clarify what they mean. Generally, a patient is regarded as constipated if they experience an infrequent passage of small, hard stools, which are difficult to pass. There is normally a wide variation in bowel habit, and not everybody opens their bowels every day. Remember to ask about the consistency as well as the frequency of motions:

- 'Are they difficult to pass?'
- 'Do they feel small and hard?'

Pain The causes of abdominal pain are legion, so keep an open mind about the source of the problem. For example, ischaemic cardiac pain and pleuritic pain can both be referred to the abdomen. Ask about the site of the pain:

- 'Is it localized or diffuse?'
- 'Does it radiate?'

- 'How long has it been there?'
- 'Has it changed in character during this time?'
- 'Is it present all the time, or does it come and go?'
- 'Does it come in spasms, or is it continuous in nature?'

Ask if there is any relationship to eating, i.e. is the pain worse when the patient is hungry or full. Does anything relieve or exacerbate the pain, such as the passing of flatus, or defaecation? Ask for any associated features of the pain such as jaundice or fever.

Anorexia True anorexia is associated with weight loss, so it is sensible to enquire about both symptoms together. It is also important to decide whether the patient has lost his/her appetite, or is afraid to eat because of pain or other symptoms. You should assess other symptoms, as anorexia can be a symptom of diseases outside the gastrointestinal tract:

- 'How is your appetite? If you were really hungry and I gave you a plate of fish and chips, would you be able to eat it?'

Patients with anorexia nervosa may deny hunger – make sure you ask about weight if the patient looks excessively thin:

- 'How would you describe your weight?'
- 'What is your ideal weight?'

Past medical history A patient with gastrointestinal disease may have a past history which includes surgery to the gastrointestinal tract: patients may present following a gastrectomy with weight loss and diarrhoea. Always enquire about any operations on the gastrointestinal tract. It is also important to enquire whether the patient has ever been jaundiced and, if so, what was the nature of the jaundice: patients may have suffered from hepatitis in the past and be unaware of the significance.

Personal and social history

It is essential to enquire how much alcohol a patient drinks. Patients often underestimate this, particularly if they consider that they may have a problem with alcohol. It is important to start cautiously with the questions:

- 'Do you drink alcohol?'
- 'How much alcohol might you drink in a week?'
- 'Is this on social occasions or are you at home?'
- 'How much alcohol may you drink at home per day?'
- 'Is that every day?'

If the patient does drink alcohol most days, enquire how long a bottle of spirits lasts, or how many bottles of wine are drunk each week. If you consider it

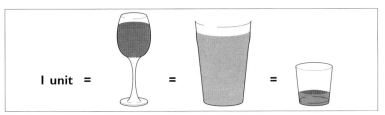

94 The unit system used to calculate alcohol intake. 1 glass of wine (0.1 litres) = 0.25 litres of beer = 1 measure of spirits (25 ml).

appropriate, enquire about the use of recreational drugs. A patient who has used recreational drugs may have been exposed to hepatitis, therefore it is important to ask him/her if he/she has ever taken any other substances (which may affect the liver). It may be worthwhile at this point explaining to the patient that the reason you are asking is purely for health reasons, as some of these drugs can affect the liver. The unit system used to calculate alcohol intake is illustrated in **94**.

Family history and treatment history

In the family history of a patient with gastrointestinal diseases it is important to know whether any close relatives have suffered from the same symptoms. Peptic ulceration often runs in families, and so does a history of alcohol abuse. It is also worth enquiring about drugs – and particularly those which may affect the liver – for example, methotrexate in the treatment of either rheumatoid arthritis or psoriasis. The patient's prescribed medications, and those bought over the counter, need to be noted with particular care in gastrointestinal problems. Such medications may also be a cause of duodenal ulceration – non-steroidal anti-inflammatory drugs (e.g. ibuprofen) or diarrhoea (antibiotics), and constipation (codeine-based analgesics).

Table 22. Examples of diferent kinds of abdominal pain

● *Gnawing pain*	Peptic ulceration
● *Colicky pain*	Associated with spasm of gallbladder or hollow viscus
● *Suprapubic pain*	Associated with urinary tract infection
● *Severe constant boring pain*	Malignancy, e.g. cancer of the pancreas

Checklist for abdominal history taking

- General approach:
    Introduce yourself.
    Establish rapport.
    Remember eye contact.

- Assess the presenting complaint (i.e. abdominal pain) and its history.
    Don't forget to ask about any history of jaundice.
    Enquire about diet.

- Ask about past medical history (particularly related to gastrointestinal disease, operations and episodes of jaundice).

- Enquire about smoking, drinking, and drugs (include in this anything about recreational drugs).

- Enquire about the social history.

- Ask about the family history (any history of peptic ulcer disease?).

- Systematic enquiry.

LISTEN TO THE ANSWERS!

Examination of the patient

Make sure that you have adequate privacy before beginning this part of the examination, and always try to preserve the patient's modesty. Ideally, for the abdominal examination patients should be exposed from the xiphisternum to the pubis, but do not leave the patient exposed for too long. Ascertain whether s/he is comfortable when lying flat with one pillow. This is the best way to assess the abdomen, but it is not always practical for some patients. Begin examining the system with the patient sitting up, and only lie them flat when you examine the abdomen itself. Remember that it may be regarded as threatening if you stand over the patient, so sit or kneel by the bedside. If you have cold hands, warm them before starting.

General observations

Begin the examination by looking at the patient's hands, then the neck, face, mouth, and upper back. During the initial assessment, look for any trace of jaundice in the skin and sclerae (95). This should be done thoroughly and quickly.

The hands Look for signs of liver disease. These include liver palms, which is

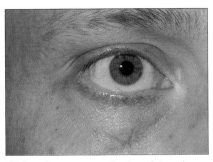

95 Jaundice, seen as yellowing of the sclera.

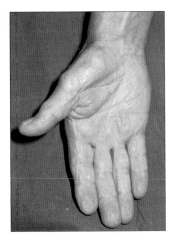

96 Dupuytren's contracture. Note tethering of the palmar skin of the ring finger.

reddening of the peripheral part of the palms due to the peripheral vasodilatation caused by oestrogen excess. Liver palms may be present in liver disease with reduced metabolism of oestrogen in the liver. They may also be found in thyrotoxicosis, pregnancy, and in users of oral contraceptives.

Dupuytren's contracture This is a flexion deformity, usually of the fourth and fifth fingers (**96**). Although there are several other causes for this condition, it may be found in liver disease and alcohol abuse.

Leuconychia This is a whitening of the nail bed caused by the hypoproteinaemia associated with liver disease.

Spider naevi These are small red vascular malformations, associated with oestrogen excess. They are easily identified because they fill from a central arteriole, and can be blanched from the middle. They are found in the distribution of the superior vena cava. A normal adult may have up to five (**105**, **106**).

Lymph nodes Examination of the cervical and axillary lymph nodes is described in Chapter 3.

Assessing the patient's nutritional status

It is always important to assess the nutritional status of a patient during the general examination. Doctors frequently fall into the trap of concentrating on specific symptoms without considering a patient's particular body habitus –

signs of weight loss associated with a malignancy may be overlooked because the doctor is focusing on abdominal pain, or the significance of obesity is not immediately recognized in the hypertensive patient. The following are simple clinical measures which can be easily undertaken to assess a patient's overall nutritional status. It is not suggested that all of these are applied on every occasion, although they are indicated in patients with cachexia or extreme obesity.

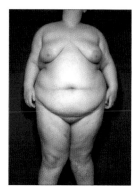

97 Morbid obesity.

Physical appearance Does the patient look extraordinarily thin or considerably overweight? Many patients have always been underweight, while others will only confirm recent weight loss if asked directly. Remember that denial is sometimes associated with anorexia nervosa. Similarly, a recent increase in weight or long-standing obesity are also of clinical significance – an explanation for the former needs to be found, while the latter is often associated with important complications such as diabetes, osteoarthritis, hypertension, and sleep apnoea. It is helpful to note your subjective impression of the patient's body habitus in the patient's case record.

Body weight and height Whenever possible, every patient should be weighed on accurate scales, and their height measured using a stadiometer. Changes in weight following treatment are essential measures of success or failure of certain therapies, e.g. weight reduction in patients with cardiac failure after commencing diuretic treatment, or weight gain following a prescription for supplemental feeds. The body mass index (BMI: weight in kg/height in metres^2) is a useful estimate of body fatness – the acceptable range is between 19 and 25 kg/m^2 with a BMI >25; 25–30 is regarded as overweight, and BMI 30 or greater is defined as obesity. A BMI >39 is indicative of extreme or 'morbid' obesity and suggests the likelihood of serious associated complications (**97**).

Regional fat distribution Epidemiological studies have confirmed that the distribution of fat within the body is also important in determining increased risk from coronary heart disease, stroke, diabetes mellitus, and hyperlipidaemia. Such an increased risk is seen in both men and women who are moderately overweight but in whom fat is deposited predominantly in the upper half of the body (upper body, truncal, or 'apple-shaped' obesity). In contrast, this is not found in overweight individuals whose fatness is largely in

Waist circumference levels

Gender	Increased risk	Substantial risk
Male	>94 cm (~37 inches)	>102 cm (~40 inches)
Female	>80 cm (~32 inches)	>88 cm (~35 inches)

the lower half of the body (lower body, gynoid, or 'pear-shaped' obesity). A simple way of assessing body fat distribution in an overweight patient is by measuring the waist circumference – there is no point in using this measure in a person who has a BMI within the acceptable range. The waist circumference is taken at the point midway between the lower border of the rib cage and the upper margin of the iliac crest.

The gender-specific waist circumference levels in the box above denote enhanced relative risk.

Skinfold thickness The measurement of skinfold thickness using skinfold callipers (usually Harpenden callipers) is an additional practical method for estimating body fatness at the bedside. The established system is to measure the skinfold thickness at four sites:

- **Triceps** is measured halfway between the acromial and olecranon processes. A fold of skin and subcutaneous tissue is pinched between your thumb and forefinger. This grip is maintained with your left hand, while the callipers are applied to the skin tuck using your right hand.
- **Biceps** skinfold thickness is measured in the same place as the triceps, but at the front of the arm with the hand supinated.
- **Subscapular** is measured at a 45° angle to the vertical at the lower of the left scapula.
- **Suprailiac** is measured in the horizontal plane, just above the iliac crest in the mid-axillary line on the left side.

Tables are available for calculating skinfold percentage fat from the sum of these four skinfolds. These measures of nutritional status should be clearly recorded in the patient's notes; it will be appropriate for them to be repeated at intervals after treatment has been commenced.

Mouth and tongue

Inspect the inside of the mouth, looking particularly at the teeth and gums. Note any obvious caries or periodontal decay and, if the patient has lost many teeth, confirm that the dentures are satisfactory. Look at the tonsils and pharynx using a light and tongue depressor if necessary. Examine the tongue, looking for smoothness (atrophy) of the papillae or soreness. Vitamin B_{12} deficiency leads to uniform atrophy of papillae over the whole tongue, which is often sore and inflamed. Other vitamin deficiency states may also cause flattening and loss of papillae including iron, nicotinic acid, pyridoxine, and folic acid. Furring of the tongue occurs in a number of acute infections and internal disorders, but is of little help with diagnosis.

Inflammation and soreness of the corners of the mouth (angular stomatitis) is seen in various deficient states, including lack of riboflavin and nicotinic acid. Most commonly, however, it results from loss of teeth or poorly fitting dentures.

Once your quick assessment of the peripheral signs is complete, proceed to examination of the abdomen. Follow the scheme: inspection, palpation, percussion, auscultation.

Inspection

Inspect the abdomen from the end of the bed, as well as from the side. Begin by looking for distension, which may be caused by masses, dilated bowel, ascites (fluid within the abdominal cavity), or enlarged organs. Take note of any visible scars or dilated subcutaneous veins. Look for signs of obvious weight loss, e.g. loose, wrinkled skin. Occasionally, dilated veins are seen radiating in all directions from the umbilicus; their appearance, which is described as a caput medusae, indicates elevation of the portal venous pressure (portal hypertension) and results from the formation of porta-systemic anastomosis via the veins in the round ligament.

Peristalsis is not normally visible except in very thin subjects. In chronic pyloric stenosis, or in intestinal obstruction, peristaltic waves may occasionally be seen.

Palpation

This is done with the right hand predominating (even if you are left-handed), with the examiner kneeling or sitting next to the patient and the arm horizontal.

Ask if the patient has any tender areas, so you can avoid these initially. Start by palpating gently in the four quadrants shown in **98**. The approximate location of the organs beneath the skin are shown in **99**. This gentle palpation should be very systematic (**100**) allowing the examiner to take note of any obvious tender areas, or masses. It is important to look at the patient's face throughout to ensure that you are not causing pain. Generalized peritonitis is obvious at this stage because it causes exquisite tenderness and a rigid abdomen.

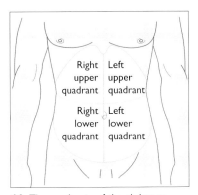

98 The quadrants of the abdomen.

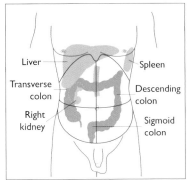

99 Approximate location of organs beneath the skin in the abdomen related to the quadrants.

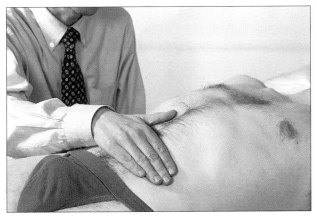

100 Begin by gentle palpation.

The liver The normal liver extends from approximately the fifth intercostal space on the right of the midline to the costal margin. It may just be palpable in the normal individual. Occasionally, it may be pushed down from above when it becomes palpable, but is still of normal size – for example, if the patient has chronic airflow limitation. This can be checked by percussing out the upper border. To feel the liver, use the flat of the hand with the fingers parallel to the costal margin. Ask the patient to take deep breaths in and out, and coordinate this with a gentle upward movement of the palpating fingertips, as the respiratory effort pushes the liver down. If the liver is enlarged, it is worth beginning the palpation in the right iliac fossa, and gradually moving the palpating hand up, coordinating this with respiration. If a liver is felt, the examiner must describe its consistency. The edge may be smooth or irregular (the latter suggesting metastases/secondary deposits), and the texture soft, firm, hard, or nodular. You should also estimate the amount of palpable liver below the costal margin in centimetres.

Occasionally, the gallbladder is felt when looking for the liver. It is a smooth round organ, arising just below the costal margin.

The spleen The normal spleen is not palpable. It lies behind the ninth rib in the left hypochondrium. It may become palpable as it enlarges; this is usually in the direction of the umbilicus. It is best palpated using the fingertips, coordinating their action with the patient's respiration. If it is not palpable with the patient lying flat, ask him/her to roll towards the examiner and advance the palpating fingers towards, and then under, the left costal margin. The left hand can be placed behind the costal margin to bring the spleen forward. Palpation of the splenic notch confirms the findings of an enlarged spleen. While the patient is in this position, percuss along the line of the seventh rib to ascertain the area of splenic dullness, thereby confirming the palpation findings.

The kidneys Palpation of the kidneys is part of the abdominal examination. In the normal individual, the lower pole of the right kidney may be felt, as it is pushed down by the liver. Examination of the kidneys is performed using both hands. To feel the left kidney, the left hand is placed behind the patient's loin, and the organ pushed forward from the back, onto the palpating right hand (**101**).

This procedure is done in reverse to feel the right kidney. The most

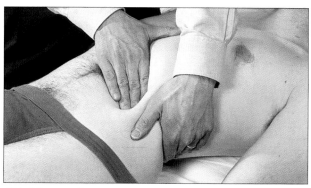

101 Palpation of the kidneys.

characteristic thing about the kidney on palpation is its mobility, in a downwards direction beneath the palpating hand.

The findings are confirmed by percussion, as the kidneys are surrounded by perinephric fat with bowel-containing gas above it, and this is resonant to percussion. The palpable left kidney is usually abnormal, except in very thin individuals. Both kidneys are situated posteriorly, and more medially than you may expect. If palpable, and enlarged, they may be ballotable. This means that a renal mass can be pushed between an anterior and a posterior palpating hand.

The bladder When this is distended it is felt as a smooth, round swelling extending upward from the pubis. The patient may experience discomfort on pressure over the area, and the swelling is typically dull to percussion. An enlarged uterus or an ovarian cyst may give rise to a swelling which is difficult to distinguish from the bladder on palpation. The distinction can be made however, if the bladder is emptied either naturally or by means of a urinary catheter.

Ascites Ascites is caused by free fluid in the abdominal cavity. It causes abdominal distension, which is often more prominent in the flanks. There are two commonly used methods of detection, percussion, and the detection of a fluid thrill. Percussion for ascites depends on eliciting shifting dullness. This is done by percussing the abdomen from the midline towards the flanks, until the note becomes dull. Keep the hand in the same position and ask the patient to roll towards you, then continue to percuss in that position. If the area where the dullness was confirmed has become resonant, this suggests free fluid in the abdominal cavity. To elicit a fluid thrill, ask an assistant to place his/her hand longitudinally along the midline. Then flick the flank beneath the area of dullness, with the other hand on the opposite side as if at the other end of a diameter of a circle (**102**). If there is a fluid thrill, it will be felt shortly after the flick, as a flutter.

Auscultation Auscultation of the normal abdomen reveals peristaltic sounds that are gurgling and bubbling in character. When the intestine is mechanically obstructed, high-pitched tinkling sounds are heard, usually in

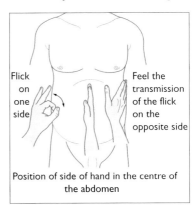

Flick on one side

Feel the transmission of the flick on the opposite side

Position of side of hand in the centre of the abdomen

102 Eliciting a fluid thrill.

association with colicky pain. In intestinal paralysis (paralytic ileus), sounds are usually absent.

When there are large amounts of fluid and gas in the stomach (or occasionally in the intestines) a splashing noise is heard when the abdomen is gently shaken. This sign is called a succussion splash: it may be normally heard if the patient has recently been eating or drinking, but is characteristically prominent in patients with delayed gastric emptying, – e.g. pyloric stenosis. Vascular sounds are sometimes heard. When there is partial obstruction of abdominal arteries, systolic murmurs may be produced and heard over the aorta, iliac arteries, or renal arteries. The latter (which are rare) may be heard over the loins.

Examination of the abdomen is not complete without examination of the external genitalia, inguinal lymph nodes, and hernial orifices (Chapter 8), followed by a rectal examination.

Rectal examination

Patients are often understandably embarrassed by this part of the examination, so it is essential to put them at their ease. Reassure the patient that although the examination may be uncomfortable and unpleasant, it should not be painful. Ask the patient to lower his/her pants to the knees, lie on his/her left side, and draw the knees up into the chest. Meanwhile, put a glove on the right hand. Lift the right buttock, with your left hand, to inspect the anus: note any sores, lesions (such as warts, or haemorrhoids), fissures, or fistulae. Place the gloved and lubricated index finger of the right hand over the anus and apply gentle pressure. The finger will be gradually admitted to the anal canal, from the front gradually backwards advancing it into the rectum. The rectal mucosa can then be felt posteriorly. The examining finger is then rotated through 360° and the mucosa felt anteriorly and laterally. Anteriorly in the male, an indentation may be felt, caused by the prostate gland. In a similar position in the female lies the cervix – a small, rounded swelling. There may be polyps (soft and attached to the rectal mucosa) or tumours (hard and irregular), but it is important to learn the difference between these pathologies and the feel of normal or constipated stool. On removing the examining finger, inspect the glove for the presence of melaena, blood, or mucus.

Illustrated physical signs

The following photographs illustrate physical signs that you may see in patients with significant liver disease.

Ascites (103) – this patient has tense, severe ascites. Severe tense swelling of the abdomen is a feature of chronic liver disease.

Hepatomegaly (104) – the large liver of this patient is indicated in the photograph. Patients with liver disease often also exhibit **spider naevi** (105 and 106).

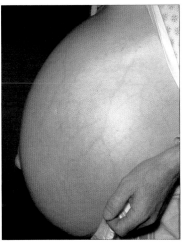

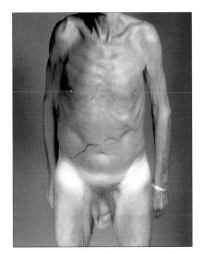

103 Ascites. Note the tense abdominal distension.

104 Hepatomegaly. The position of the liver is indicated.

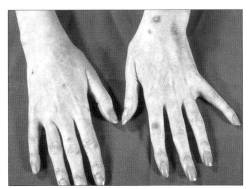

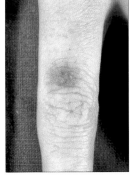

105 and 106 Spider naevi in patient with liver disease.

Table 23. Findings in a normal abdominal examination

- Start by assessing the patient's hands, but don't take too long. Also look at cervical and axillary adenopathy and signs of abdominal disease in the face
- Expose the patient from the xiphisternum to the pubis
- Ask the patient to identify tender areas, and palpate superficially over the whole abdomen
- Use deep palpation looking for liver, spleen and kidneys
- Percuss over palpated areas
- Look for hernias and lymph nodes
- Auscultate over the aorta and renal arteries
- Mention a rectal examination

Table 24. Care of the patient with gastrointestinal disease

- Ensure that adults are able to feed themselves
- Ensure that patients are able to use a commode and/or a bedpan
- Keep stool/vomit charts as necessary: observation of colour, consistency, amount, and odour of stool
- Assess the dietary needs of patients

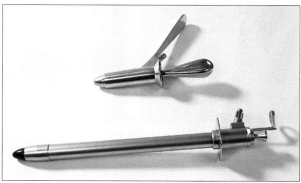

107 A proctoscope (top) and sigmoidoscope.

Therapeutic and technical skills

Proctoscopy and sigmoidoscopy

If the patient has a normal rectal examination, but you suspect a lesion higher up, it is important to proceed to proctoscopy and sigmoidoscopy.

The proctoscope and sigmoidoscope are illustrated in **107**. Disposable versions made of plastic are available for single use; the reusable kind are metal. Make sure you have an operating light source before beginning the procedure.

Liver biopsy

This used to be a procedure performed by junior doctors, but because of the high incidence of adverse events, it is now frequently performed using ultrasound imaging. It is contraindicated if the platelet count is less than 80×10^9/L, or the International Normalized Ratio (INR) is greater than 1.3 (this can be corrected by giving vitamin K). As a precaution, make sure that the patient's serum has been saved for cross-matching. After the procedure, the patient must lie on his/her right side for four hours, and pulse and blood pressure should be measured half-hourly.

Sigmoidoscopy

- Wear gloves as for the rectal examination, and if you are wearing a tie, tuck it into your shirt.

- The patient should be in the left lateral position, with the knees drawn up, and the buttocks at the edge of the couch. Warn that you are going to pass an instrument, which may feel cold and uncomfortable, into the rectum.

- Check that the components of the sigmoidoscope or proctoscope are all present, functional, and fit together correctly before you start.

- Slide the lubricated instrument into the anus, with the end directed towards the pubic symphysis.

- Detach and remove the obturator, and connect the light source.

- Inflate the rectum manually, using the rubber bulb, and guide the instrument under direct vision to the rectosigmoid junction, and beyond if possible.

- The normal rectal mucosa is smooth and glistening, and should not bleed on contact.

- Biopsies can be taken of abnormal looking areas, or normal ones if sub-acute inflammation is suspected.

Proctoscopy

This is similar to sigmoidoscopy, but a slightly easier procedure to perform.

● The proctoscope is passed in the same way, towards the symphysis pubis, the obturator is removed, and the light source attached.

● The proctoscope is removed as the patient pushes down.

● Haemorrhoids (distended veins), and local anal conditions such as fissures can be visualized.

Upper gastrointestinal endoscopy

This is performed by a specially trained operator (either medical or nursing), and is done as a day case or outpatient procedure. The patient is fasted overnight. Informed consent to the procedure must be obtained beforehand.

● The patient is asked to lie in the left lateral position, and the back of the throat sprayed with local anaesthetic.

● If the patient is particularly anxious, intravenous sedation may be necessary (a benzodiazepine is usually used). If s/he has had previous respiratory problems, nasal oxygen may be necessary.

● The endoscopist aims the endoscope at the back of the throat, and passes the tube down the oesophagus under direct vision.

● The lining of the stomach and duodenum are visualized. The mucosa should have a glistening appearance, and any abnormal areas should be biopsied.

● After the procedure, the patient should remain nil-by-mouth for about 1–2 hours. If he/she has had intravenous sedation, he/she must be accompanied home.

Nasogastric tube

This is a simple, but unpleasant procedure for the patient. It can be messy, so wear gloves. The cooperative patient is asked to sit upright.

● A well-lubricated nasogastric tube (**108**) is then inserted into the nose and advanced along the base of the nasal cavity until it reaches the back of the patient's throat. This makes most normal patients gag.

● The patient is then asked to swallow hard – this may be helped by giving him/her a glass of water.

● As the patient swallows, the tube is advanced down the oesophagus towards the stomach. The tube has 10 cm marks on it to show how far it has been advanced; the stomach should be at a distance of 40 cm from the mouth.

● Proof that the tube is in the stomach is gained by aspirating the tube and testing the aspirate for acid, with litmus paper.

● If you are in doubt about its position, ask for a chest X-ray; the tube has a radio-opaque line, and so can be easily seen on the film.

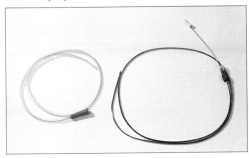

108 A nasogastric tube.

Abdominal paracentesis

This procedure is performed to drain ascites. It can be done as a diagnostic or therapeutic manoeuvre. Ask the patient to empty his/her bladder before you begin.

● Lie the patient supine, and percuss the lower abdomen to check the extent of the ascitic dullness.

● Clean the lower abdomen with iodine or a similar antiseptic solution. Infiltrate an area as shown in **109**, between McBurney's point and the umbilicus, taking care to miss the inferior epigastric artery, which runs under the rectus sheath.

● Always aspirate before injecting the local anaesthetic, to ensure that you have not entered a blood vessel. While leaving time for the local anaesthetic to work, wash your hands, and put on sterile gloves.

● For a diagnostic tap, insert a 21-gauge (green) needle at this point, and aspirate. For drainage, use a suprapubic or peritoneal dialysis catheter.

● The catheter comes with a trocar, which has a sharp point. Penetrate the skin with this, and once ascitic fluid appears, carefully advance the catheter, and remove the trocar.

● Attach the end to a sterile drainage bag with an adjustable valve, and make sure that the fluid does not drain too fast, as this can cause systemic hypotension. Ideally, drain approximately 3 litres per day. Secure the catheter with tape, giving some room for movement.

● As the fluid drains, the flow may become positional, so if the tube appears to be blocked, moving the patient may solve the problem.

Samples from either a diagnostic or therapeutic tap should be sent to microbiology for culture, including acid-fast bacilli (AFB), chemistry for glucose and protein, and cytology for identification of the cells.

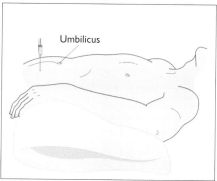

109 Abdominal paracentesis.

Key laboratory tests

Liver function tests Liver function is measured by an assessment of hepatic enzymes, alkaline phosphatase (ALP), aspartate amino transferase (AST) or alanine amino transferase (ALT) and gamma-glutamyl transferase (γGT), together with albumin, bilirubin, and total serum protein. The bilirubin, AST and ALP are all moderately elevated in hepatocellular jaundice. The ALP is highly elevated in obstructive jaundice – often out of all proportion to the other two enzymes. In this situation there is usually a corresponding increase in the γGT. γGT is more specifically elevated in alcoholic liver disease – and suggests the presence of excess alcohol, particularly if the other enzymes are normal or mildly raised. The albumin is a measure of hepatic synthetic function, and is a useful marker of the severity of hepatic impairment. Albumin is characteristically reduced in chronic liver disease, whereas the total serum protein level is usually increased.

Clotting Clotting is measured by estimating the prothrombin time (PT or INR), the partial thromboplastin time (PTTK) and the thrombin time (TT). Prothrombin time provides an estimate of the performance of the extrinsic and common coagulation pathways. The PTTK is also prolonged in abnormalities of either the intrinsic or common pathways. The TT measures the transformation of prothrombin to thrombin. It is prolonged by fibrinogen deficiency. Recently, the coagulation cascade has been reinvestigated with the discovery of protein C, protein S and anti-thrombin III. Deficiencies of those factors should be sought in patients with a hypercoagulable state.

Hepatitis B serology The serological markers of hepatitis B are important in the assessment of the relative infection risk of carriers. In a patient incubating hepatitis B, or with an acute attack, there are positive tests for HbsAg (surface antigen) and HbeAg (a marker of high infectivity). The patient may also have the antibodies anti-Hbc, IgG, and IgM. In the carrier state, HbsAg is positive. HbeAg is either positive or negative, depending on whether the patient is highly (positive HbeAg) or not very highly (negative HbeAg) infectious. In the convalescence phase of an acute attack the surface (HbsAg) and e antigen (HbeAg) are negative, but anti-Hbs and anti-Hbi antibodies become positive. After successful vaccination, the patient is positive for anti-Hbs only.

The following figures demonstrate the features required to make a diagnosis of common gastrointestinal and genitourinary diseases: peptic ulceration (**110**), large bowel carcinoma (**111**), inflammatory bowel disease (**112**), chronic liver disease (**113**), chronic renal failure (**114**), and urinary tract infection (**115**).

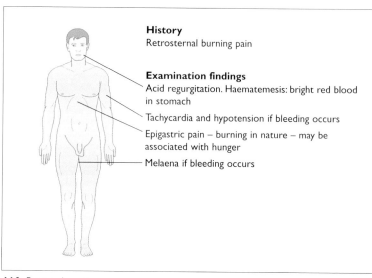

History
Retrosternal burning pain

Examination findings
Acid regurgitation. Haematemesis: bright red blood in stomach

Tachycardia and hypotension if bleeding occurs

Epigastric pain – burning in nature – may be associated with hunger

Melaena if bleeding occurs

110 Peptic ulceration.

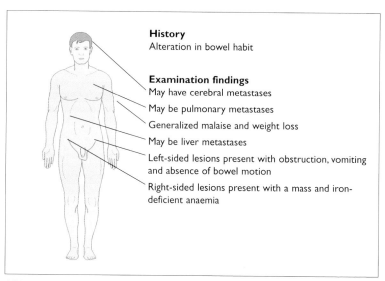

History
Alteration in bowel habit

Examination findings
May have cerebral metastases

May be pulmonary metastases

Generalized malaise and weight loss

May be liver metastases

Left-sided lesions present with obstruction, vomiting and absence of bowel motion

Right-sided lesions present with a mass and iron-deficient anaemia

111 Large bowel carcinoma.

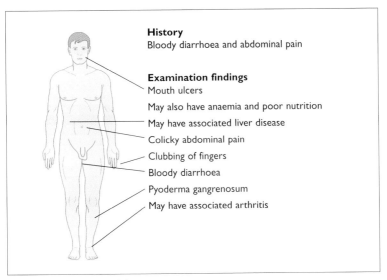

History
Bloody diarrhoea and abdominal pain

Examination findings
Mouth ulcers

May also have anaemia and poor nutrition

May have associated liver disease

Colicky abdominal pain

Clubbing of fingers

Bloody diarrhoea

Pyoderma gangrenosum

May have associated arthritis

112 Inflammatory bowel disease.

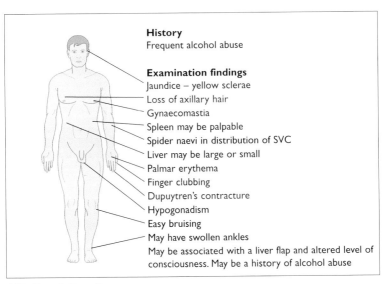

History
Frequent alcohol abuse

Examination findings
Jaundice – yellow sclerae

Loss of axillary hair

Gynaecomastia

Spleen may be palpable

Spider naevi in distribution of SVC

Liver may be large or small

Palmar erythema

Finger clubbing

Dupuytren's contracture

Hypogonadism

Easy bruising

May have swollen ankles

May be associated with a liver flap and altered level of consciousness. May be a history of alcohol abuse

113 Chronic liver disease.

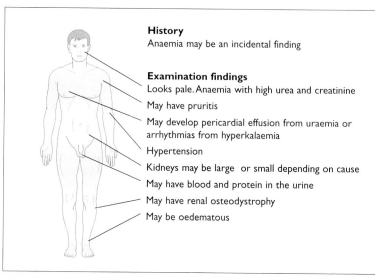

History
Anaemia may be an incidental finding

Examination findings
Looks pale. Anaemia with high urea and creatinine

May have pruritis

May develop pericardial effusion from uraemia or arrhythmias from hyperkalaemia

Hypertension

Kidneys may be large or small depending on cause

May have blood and protein in the urine

May have renal osteodystrophy

May be oedematous

114 Chronic renal failure.

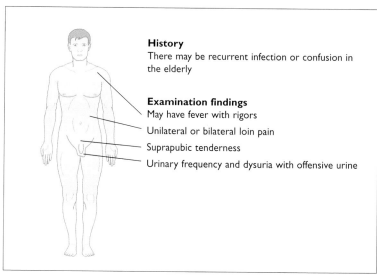

History
There may be recurrent infection or confusion in the elderly

Examination findings
May have fever with rigors

Unilateral or bilateral loin pain

Suprapubic tenderness

Urinary frequency and dysuria with offensive urine

115 Urinary tract infection.

5 The locomotor system

Locomotor disorders are one of the most common causes of pain and disability, both in hospital and within the community. Almost everyone has had some time off work with back pain during their career, or has suffered a similar minor locomotor problem. Examination of the locomotor system is quite difficult, particularly as it is somewhat diverse – the high prevalence of rheumatic conditions in the general population is not reflected by the quality of rheumatological examination in practice. Conditions affecting the locomotor system are diverse, and range from very minor soft tissue conditions such as tennis elbow to very severe, life-threatening connective tissue diseases, such as systemic lupus erythematosus (SLE). This requires history taking and examination to be extremely flexible, allowing for a quick 'spot' diagnosis, or to give time and understanding to patients with more complex problems where necessary.

Applied anatomy and physiology of the joints

The locomotor system is made up of muscles and joints. The two basic structures of joints which permit mobility are cartilage and fibrous tissue. Cartilaginous joints are those in which a wide range of movement is required. The anatomy of the synovial joint is shown in **116**.

In a **fibrous joint,** there is less mobility and therefore the joint is simpler in structure and associated with fewer medical problems.

In a **synovial joint,** the bony ends are covered by hyaline cartilage and surrounded by a capsule. The inside of the capsule is covered by a synovial membrane which has secretory and absorptive tissue. The synovial membrane produces synovial fluid by ultrafiltration.

In addition to joints, there are several other fluid-filled sacs within the body known as bursae. These can also become inflamed and symptomatic.

The joints are moved by the actions of muscles, which are attached to bone by tendons. The two main causes

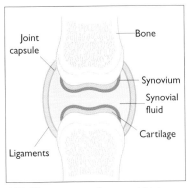

116 The anatomy of a synovial joint.

of arthritis or joint disease are degenerative change and inflammatory change.

- Degenerative change is seen in patients with osteoarthritis in whom the cartilage layers have become thinned and fibrillated and thus degenerate, giving rise to symptoms.
- Inflammatory joint disease occurs in patients in whom there is synovitis, or inflammation of the synovium, causing joint inflammation and thus secondary damage to the joint.

Tendons, ligaments and fascial structures attach to the periosteum by a specialized structure, the enthesis, and this can become inflamed, causing an enthesitis, e.g. plantar faciitis.

Assessment and diagnosis of joint disease

Assessment of a patient with disease of the musculoskeletal system involves an assessment not only of the history of his/her symptoms, but also of the degree of disability and handicap.

Taking the history

The cardinal symptoms of joint disease are pain, stiffness, swelling, deformity, disability, and systemic illness. It is often the history and the pattern of joint involvement that lead to the diagnosis of the rheumatic condition.

For example, a symmetrical polyarthritis which is inflammatory and mainly affects small joints is called rheumatoid arthritis.

The presenting complaint

Pain Pain is the most common reason for a rheumatological consultation, but it is often quite a vague symptom and requires specific questioning. The degree of pain does not relate directly to the severity of the condition. Although open questions are essential to start the consultation, a question such as: 'Where is

Locomotor history taking

A locomotor history allows the doctor to answer the four following questions and thus make a diagnosis:

- Is the patient's problem caused by a symmetrical or an asymmetrical arthritis?
- Is it a monoarthritis, or does it affect several joints – a polyarthritis?
- Is it an inflammatory or a non-inflammatory arthritis?
- Does it affect large joints or small joints?

the pain?' may get a vague answer. Thus, it is important to use focused and closed questions, and also to ask the patient to point not only to the general area of the pain but also to the place where the pain is at its maximum intensity:

- 'Where do you get the pain?'
- 'Does it go anywhere else?'
- 'Show me the worst spot.'
- 'Does it go down your arms or legs?'

As some arthritic conditions such as a prolapsed intervertebral disc may cause nerve root irritation, the pain may be in a dermatome distribution and quite distant from the original problem. Rheumatological pain is also referred; for example, shoulder pain is felt in the upper arm, and hip pain is felt in the knee. It is important also to enquire whether the pain is associated with other symptoms of locomotor problems such as stiffness and swelling.

Locomotor pain is often related to movement, and it is important to enquire whether the pain gets better with rest, or improves with increased activity. Pain that gets better with activity or as the day progresses, is more likely to be due to inflammation. Pain that gets worse during the day is likely to be due to degenerative change:

- 'When is the pain at its worst?'
- 'Does it get better or worse during the day?'

Most locomotor system pain is better at night; however, pain from severe arthritis and also malignant disease keeps the patient awake. Night pain is likely to suggest a more significant problem, like a hip that needs replacing or a disease with a poorer prognosis. Some locomotor system pain is caused by fairly specific abnormalities, such as tennis elbow. In these patients the pain is very specific and is localized to one particular spot. The patient can often show the exact spot:

- 'Can you find the exact spot?'

Some patients have a lot of non-specific aches and pains which may have a non-organic cause. This is often called arthralgia. It is important to exclude organic causes before reassuring the patient that nothing is seriously amiss.

Stiffness Patients with locomotor system problems often complain of stiffness. This is an inability to get the joints moving again after a period of rest. In inflammatory conditions this stiffness is much worse in the mornings and gradually wears off over a period of one or two hours. The length of time that the stiffness lasts is related to the severity of the inflammation. Patients with degenerative change also have stiffness, but the stiffness is related to inactivity, and tends to come on when sitting down for a period of ten minutes or longer.

The stiffness usually takes less than half an hour to resolve, but is worse as the day progresses:
- 'Do you feel stiff?'
- 'When?'
- 'How long does it take you to get going when you get up in the morning?'

Swelling In patients with joint pain and stiffness, it is important to enquire about local swelling. Swelling may be symmetrical or asymmetrical, depending on the kind of arthritis and is of three kinds:
- **Synovial swelling:** this feels soft and 'boggy', and is associated with heat and local inflammation. It is often symmetrical and is associated with inflammatory conditions.
- **Bony swelling:** this is associated with degenerative conditions and causes joint deformity, but little associated heat and redness. It has often been present for longer than soft tissue swelling.
- **Fluctuant swelling:** this is caused by fluid and may feel hot, but is not compressible. It is important to ask the patient whether the swollen joint is hot and red, and whether the swelling is there permanently or whether it comes and goes.
- Ask: 'Do your joints swell? Which joints are affected? Do they feel hot to the touch? Do they go red?'

Deformity Deformity is often the end result of an arthritic process. You should enquire over what period of time the deformity has been developing, and the association of the deformity with swelling and pain:
- 'How long has this been going on?'

Disability Disability is frequently the result of an arthritic process. In the history, you should estimate how much the patient is able to do and how much the disease interferes with his/her day-to-day life. The sort of questions you will need to ask will depend on the patient's daily activity and whether he/she can carry out their normal job. For example, a tennis elbow or a frozen shoulder may be severely disabling in somebody who needs to use their upper limb (a librarian, a painter, or a secretary), while painful feet are a serious disability in a postman. It is a useful exercise to ask the patient to take you through an average day – and enquire how he/she does things like shopping or cooking – and whether he/she has help from other people or uses appliances.

Systemic illness Connective tissue diseases, which are multisystem diseases, may present with locomotor system problems. It is therefore important to ask patients whether they have noticed fever, weight loss, a tendency to fatigue, and

Table 25. Examples of different kinds of joint swelling

- *Synovitis*   'Boggy', symmetrical swelling which feels hot
- *Osteoarthritis* Hard, bony swelling which generally feels cool
- *Fluid*   Soft, fluctuant swelling which feels hot

lethargy. In addition, there may have been a problem with rashes, particularly the photosensitive rash of SLE.

In general, although locomotor system problems are rarely life-threatening, they may cause significant disability in those who suffer them, and are frequently associated with subclinical symptoms of depression. You should enquire whether the patient has suffered from feelings of depression, excessive tiredness, and weepiness. These may be part of a primary problem, or they may have developed secondary to the locomotor system problem.

Past history

Rheumatological complaints may have a long history, so it is important to establish whether there is any locomotor system problem in the past medical history.

For example, a patient with generalized osteoarthritis may have a problem with one large joint affected by osteoarthritis, and may also have had evidence of cervical spondylosis in the past. The patients may feel that this new pain is part of a different condition. You must establish whether there has been a history of acute injury or damage to a particular joint. This is important in osteoarthritis where mechanical damage may predispose to the condition; for example, footballers are likely to get osteoarthritis of the knee. In the inflammatory arthritides it is important to enquire about associated conditions such as iritis.

Personal and social history

Some occupations predispose to specific problems: for example, dentists may develop osteoarthritis of the neck due to their working position, and dancers may develop osteoarthritis of the feet. Leisure activities can also predispose to osteoarthritis, and you should enquire about particularly violent types of physical exercise.

Table 26. Important areas of enquiry

- Pain
- Stiffness
- Swelling
- Deformity
- Disability
- Systemic illness

There are some specific occupational rheumatic diseases which have now become common parlance – for example, housemaid's knee (pre-patella bursitis), tennis elbow (lateral epicondylitis), and weaver's bottom (ischial bursitis).

Family and treatment history

There is an inherited component to inflammatory musculoskeletal diseases such as rheumatoid arthritis and ankylosing spondylitis, so you should enquire about any familial history of inflammatory arthritis. Recent research in twins has suggested that osteoarthritis also runs in families. However, many patients may remember that their grandparents had rheumatism but cannot recall the diagnosis. It may be helpful to ask the patient to describe the abnormalities he/she remembers, as well as to tell you what he/she thinks was wrong. You need to enquire about drugs such as aspirin and non-steroidal anti-inflammatory drugs, not only to assess their efficacy but also to assess their side-effects (in particular gastric irritation and gastrointestinal bleeding). Patients with rheumatoid arthritis are particularly prone to this. Remember also that several patients with inflammatory arthritic conditions may be on long-term steroid therapy and have associated side-effects.

Finally, it is important not to forget that some connective tissue diseases can be drug-induced. Beware the patient with SLE who has been taking long-term phenothiazines for a psychiatric condition, and who has developed the condition as a consequence of the drug intake.

Checklist for rheumatological history taking

- General approach, establish rapport, eye contact.

- Assess the patient's complaint, particularly with relation to pain.

- Ask about past medical history of rheumatic problems.

- Take a detailed drug history of drugs which may precipitate and be used to treat the condition.

- Ask about social and occupational history.

- Ask about family history; remember that several rheumatic problems are inherited.

- Systematic enquiry.

LISTEN TO THE ANSWERS !

Examination of the patient

Examination of the locomotor system can be complicated, so for the purpose of this book a rheumatological screen will be described, followed by a simple system for examining other joints. The screen is known as the (GALS) Locomotor System Screen (see right).

The locomotor system screen

- G = Look at the **G**ait
- A = **A**rms
- L = **L**egs
- S = **S**pine

General observations

Gait Observe the patient from the front and sides while he/she is standing in his/her underwear (**117, 118**), looking for any kind of asymmetry and deformity such as one leg shorter or longer (**119**) than the other, or abnormality of the spinal curvature (kyphosis, scoliosis, or a loss of lumbar lordosis). Observe the patient walking to make sure that the gait is normal, that he/she is swinging the arms and moving the legs symmetrically. Look out for an antalgic gait, and make sure that both the knees are straight. An antalgic gait is an abnormality of gait rhythm, where the patient avoids bearing weight on the painful leg and spends most of the gait cycle on the unaffected limb. This may suggest a problem in hip, knee, hindfoot, midfoot, or forefoot.

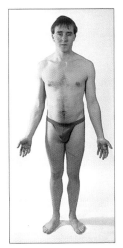

117 Look at the patient from the front.

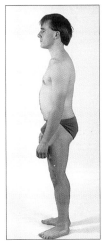

118 Look at the patient from the side.

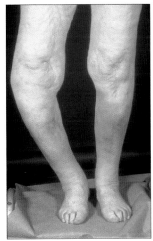

119 Paget's disease of the tibia (a sabre tibia) and secondary osteoarthritis of the knee.

Examination of the arms (1)

During the general inspection you should inspect for abnormalities such as swelling or deformity, and look for any skin changes which may be associated with arthritis, for example, digital vasculitis in SLE, or evidence of peripheral infarcts from Raynaud's phenomenon.

● Ask the patient to show you his/her hands, palms down, then turn them over – this is an assessment of the radioulnar joint, which is a common site for rheumatoid arthritis (**120**). Remember to keep the elbows tucked in, or patients can use their shoulders to perform this movement.

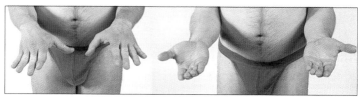

120 Assessment of radioulnar joint movement.

● Ask the patient to make a tight fist with each hand (**121**); this is a position of function of the hands, and you can also assess power grip.

● Ask the patient to place the tip of each finger onto the tip of the thumb in turn (**122**); this permits an assessment of the dexterity and fine movement of the hand, which is limited in rheumatoid arthritis.

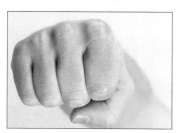
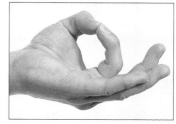

121 Ask the patient to make a fist. **122** Opposition of the thumb.

Examination of the arms (2)

● Squeeze across from the second to the fifth metacarpals (**123**); this is an assessment of joint tenderness. Tenderness across the metacarpophalangeal joints is a sign of rheumatoid arthritis.

● Next, ask the patient to put his/her hands behind the head, pressing the shoulders right back; this is an assessment of abduction and external rotation of the shoulder with flexion of the elbow (**124**). It is a measurement of shoulder and elbow movement as well of function; it is not possible to put on a tie or comb your hair unless you can do this manoeuvre.

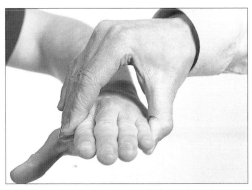

123 Assessment of metacarpophalangeal tenderness.

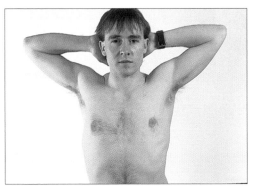

124 Assessment of abduction and external rotation of the shoulders.

Examination of the legs

• Ask the patient to lie back on the couch and flex the hip and knee while holding the knee. Ensure normal knee flexion, feel for crepitus, and also test hip flexion.

• Then passively and internally rotate the hip with the knee and hip still flexed (**125**); this is a measurement of knee movement, and internal rotation of the hip.

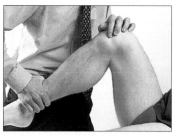

125 Assessment of knee flexion and hip internal rotation.

• Ask the patient to flex, extend, invert, and evert the ankle in order to assess tibiotalar (affected by osteoarthritis) and subtalar (affected by inflammatory arthritis) movements (**126**, **127**).

• Squeeze the metatarsals, again looking for rheumatoid arthritis in the same way as looking over the metacarpals.

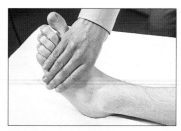

126 Assess tibiotalar movement.

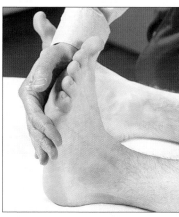

127 Assess subtalar movement.

Examination of the spine

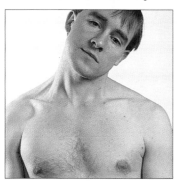

128 Assessment of lateral flexion of the neck.

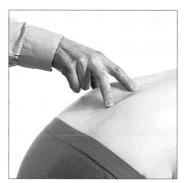

129 A modification of the Schober's test for spinal movement.

- Ask the patient to stand up and to put his/her ear on to each shoulder in turn; this is an assessment of lateral flexion of the neck (**128**) which is lost with either osteoarthritis or rheumatoid arthritis affecting the neck.

- Put two fingers over adjacent spinous processes in the lumbar region and then ask the patient to bend over and touch his/her toes; your fingers should move apart. This is a modification of a Schober's test which is designed to pick up a lack of movement associated with ankylosing spondylitis (**129**).

Regional joint examination

Low back pain   The lumbar spine should be examined with the patient standing, supine, and prone:

- With the patient standing, assess the curvature of the spine. Scoliosis may be due to muscle spasm in acute sciatica or may be postural in leg length inequality. Loss of the normal lordosis is a sign of inflammatory spinal disease, such as ankylosing spondylitis.
- Palpate the erector spinae muscles to assess spasm.
- Perform a modified Schober's test (see above).
- Ask the patient to lean over to each side in turn and run his/her hand down the side of the leg to the knee; this assesses lateral flexion.
- Then ask the patient to lean over backwards to assess extension. If extension is painful, facet joint disease (usually degenerative) may be present.

With the patient supine on the couch, assess straight leg raising:

- Lift the leg by placing your hand underneath the ankle and passively flex the hip, keeping the knee extended. When the limit is reached, perform the sciatic stretch test by passively dorsiflexing the ankle. The test assesses irritation of the low lumbar and upper sacral nerve roots. If the patient complains of sensory disturbance (pains, pins and needles, or numbness) anywhere below the knee, then the test is positive.
- Now ask the patient to turn over, remove the pillow from the head of the couch and place it under the pelvis and abdomen. This slightly flexes the lumbar spine and is a comfortable position for the patient. Palpate down the spinous processes in turn and along the erector spinae muscles, looking for tenderness.
- Then perform the femoral stretch test. This is the counterpart to the sciatic stretch test and assesses irritation in the upper lumbar nerve roots, which contribute to the femoral nerve. Passively flex the knee and, holding the foot, gently extend the hip. If this provokes spasm of the quadriceps and the patient complains of sensory disturbance over the front of the thigh, then the test is positive.

Hip pain Hip joint disease produces pain in the groin which may radiate down the anterior thigh to the knee. Pain over the lateral pelvis and thigh is more likely to be due to trochanteric bursitis, and pain in the buttock may be due to ischial bursitis, sacroiliitis, or lumbar spine disease.

- To assess the hip joints, ask the patient to lie supine on the couch. Look for flexion deformity at the hip. The hip joints are deep and cannot be directly palpated. Assess flexion at the hip with the knee flexed to relax the hamstrings.
- Then assess internal and external rotation in flexion. Internal rotation is frequently restricted early in hip disease. Place the hip in the neutral position, extend the knee, and abduct and adduct the hip in turn. Extension is assessed by either hanging the leg over the side of the couch or with the patient in the prone position.

Knee pain Ensure the patient is sitting propped up on the couch with the knees extended and the legs relaxed. Look for flexion deformity and for valgus and varus deformities.

- Look at the quadriceps muscles, which may be wasted in significant knee disease.
- Look for swelling. A large effusion will cause obvious suprapatellar swelling. Depress the patella with your fingertips: when the pressure is released, it will bounce up (the 'patella tap') if a large effusion is present.

- A small effusion may be detected by the 'bulge' test. To perform this test, empty the hollow next to the medial aspect of the patella by stroking it firmly and then push with the flat of your hand against the lateral aspect of the knee. If the medial hollow becomes filled in by a bulge, then an effusion is present (the normal knee contains only 1–2 ml of fluid, and this is insufficient to cause a bulge). Palpate the popliteal fossa for swelling, which is most often due to a Baker's cyst.
- Flex and extend the knee to its fullest extent in either direction, with your hand placed on the knee to feel for crepitus. Look for hyperextension, which is a feature of hypermobility syndrome and is commonly associated with mechanical knee pain.
- Assess stability of the knee by attempting to distract the knee first medially and then laterally while holding the knee in a few degrees of flexion. If there is abnormal movement then the collateral ligaments are lax.

Shoulder pain   The shoulder is a complex structure and shoulder pain may have many causes. Pain from the glenohumeral joint (the shoulder joint proper) radiates to the front and side of the upper arm. Pain over the top of the shoulder suggests acromioclavicular joint disease, and this may be confirmed by point tenderness over the joint and pain on forced extension of the shoulder.

- With the patient sitting and facing you, observe the shoulders for asymmetry and swelling. Effusions point anteriorly.
- Palpate the capsule over the anterior humeral head and the supraspinatus tendon over the lateral upper humerus for tenderness.
- Assess flexion, extension, abduction, adduction, and internal and external rotation both actively and passively.

In glenohumeral joint disease, such as adhesive capsulitis and rheumatoid arthritis (degenerative disease of this joint is not common), passive and active movements will be equally restricted. In contrast, disease of the rotator cuff, such as calcific tendinitis and degenerative rupture, causes restricted active movements, but passive movements remain full. Painful arc syndrome is a feature of rotator cuff disease affecting the supraspinatus component. It is detected by asking the patient to hold his/her arms up above the head, close to the ears, with the palms turned outwards (that is, with the shoulders internally rotated) and then asking him/her to lower the arms slowly sideways. Increased pain, due to compression of the inflamed tendon between the acromion and the rotating humeral head, occurs at some point with the arc of movement.

Pain in the hand and wrist The hand is examined in some detail in the GALS screen (see above). The following should be noted in addition. When examining the hands, stand in front of the patient and examine both hands at the same time, comparing the two sides. When you ask the patient to hold out his/her hands, make sure that the hands are held free of the knees, and the fingers spread. Unless this is done, you will miss minor degrees of flexion deformity of the fingers and the dropped fingers characteristic of extensor tendon rupture. Pain in the fingers may be due to osteoarthritis; look for bony swellings on the distal interphalangeal joints (Heberden's nodes) and on the proximal interphalangeal joints (Bouchard's nodes). Pronounced soft tissue swelling of these joints indicates inflammatory arthritis. Severe inflammatory arthrides, such as rheumatoid or psoriatic arthritis, with marked bone loss may lead to 'telescoping' of the fingers with redundancy of the soft tissues and to flail joints, which have lost all integrity. A combination of fixed joints (due to bony ankylosis) and flail joints is a feature of psoriatic arthritis.

Examination of the hand is not complete without an assessment of function. Hand the patient a pen and ask him/her to write, ask the patient to do up and undo buttons, and to hold a cup and bring it to his/her lips.

Should you find specific abnormalities in the locomotor system using this system, you should then do a regional joint examination remembering the mnemonic look, feel, move:

- **Look** for swelling and deformity.
- **Feel** to see whether the swelling is hot and symmetrical.
- Then **move** the joint.

Don't worry if you can't remember the range of movement of all joints as you may compare this either with the patient – who may have a normal joint on the other side – or with your own joints.

Recording a normal locomotor system examination
Examination findings are recorded as shown in **Table 27**.

Illustrated physical signs
The following photographs illustrate some common locomotor system abnormalities.

Rheumatoid hands (**130**): note the symmetrical small joint polyarthritis with ulnar deviation and swan-neck deformities.

Osteoarthritis of the hands (**131**): note the squaring of the hand caused

Table 27. Recording a normal locomotor system examination

GALS		Appearance	Movement
G	Gait	✔	✔
A	Arms	✔	✔
L	Legs	✔	✔
S	Spine	✔	✔

by first carpometacarpal (CMC) involvement and distal interphalangeal involvement.

Gout of the great toe (132): This photograph is characteristic of acute gout. Scleroderma causes characteristic skin thickening (133), while systemic lupus erythematosus (SLE) causes a photosensitive rash in a characteristic butterfly distribution (134).

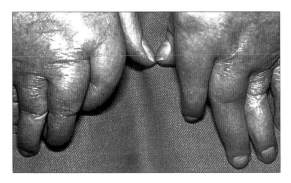

130 Rheumatoid hands with swelling and swan neck deformities.

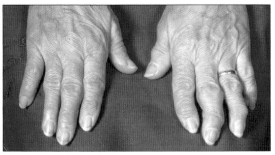

131 Osteoarthritis of the hands with squaring at the first CMC and Heberden's nodes.

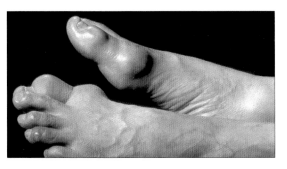

132 Gout of the great toe. Note the erythema and swelling.

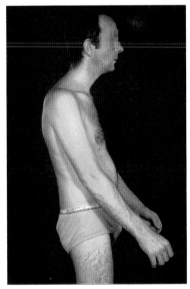

133 Scleroderma of the hands. Note the tight, shiny skin.

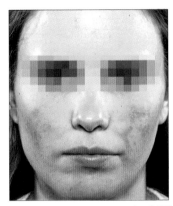

134 The photosensitive rash of SLE.

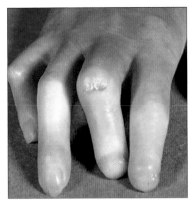

135 Ankylosing spondylitis.

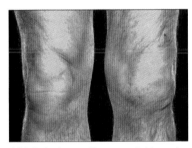

136 Baker's cyst (front view). Note the swollen left knee.

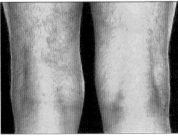

137 Baker's cyst (back view). Note the fusiform swelling on the left.

Ankylosing spondylitis causes characteristics changes in posture (135), and arthritis of the knee (136) may rupture into the calf (137).

Therapeutic and interventional skills

Aspiration of the knee (aseptic technique)

Warn the patient that this is a rather unpleasant procedure, but that it should not be more painful than having blood taken. Make sure that the patient is relaxed and lying on the couch with the knee slightly flexed, sometimes a pillow or a rolled up towel behind the knee is helpful.

Aspiration can be carried out from either the medial or lateral compartment; however, it is slightly easier on the medial side, provided that no osteophytes are present.

● Palpate the outline of the patella and the medial joint line. Imagine that these two structures form a 'T'.

● Before beginning, it is kinder – but not absolutely necessary – to infiltrate the area with local anaesthetic at the aspiration site. Use 1 ml of 1% lignocaine (xylocaine); remember always to aspirate before injecting. If you do this before preparing your aspiration needle the preparation time allows the local anaesthetic some time to work (about 5 min).

● Prepare a 20-ml syringe (or larger for a larger effusion) with a 21-gauge (green) needle, and a sterile specimen container for the aspirate.

● Insert the needle at an angle of approximately 45° in the gap between the lower border of the patella and the medial joint line. When the needle is in the joint space, synovial fluid should be aspirated freely.

● Continue to aspirate the joint fluid by changing the syringe when it is full. If you are injecting with steroid, this can be done at the end of the aspiration procedure through the same needle.

Fortunately, the synovium has antibacterial properties, so it is unlikely that you will cause a septic arthritis. However, it is important to be careful about using a 'no-touch' technique when aspirating joints, as septic arthritis is a potential disaster. Following the aspiration and or injection it is necessary to warn a patient to rest the knee for 24–48 hours. The pain may also be worse for the first day or so before improving.

Key laboratory tests
Erythrocyte sedimentation rate (ESR) The ESR is a non-specific test of inflammation and is often raised in inflammatory locomotor system disease.

You need to be a little cautious about its interpretation, as intercurrent infections can cause the level to be elevated.

The rheumatoid factor This is positive in the majority of patients with rheumatoid arthritis. However, rheumatoid disease can be present with a negative rheumatoid factor. This emphasizes that rheumatoid arthritis is a clinical diagnosis.

Anti-nuclear antibodies These antibodies are positive in patients with connective tissue diseases. Patients with SLE may also have a high circulating level of anti-DNA or SM antibodies. Patients with other connective tissue diseases may have high levels of extractable nuclear antigens (ENA). The antibodies are helpful in predicting the pattern of involvement of the disease, and therefore the outcome.

Table 28. Care of the patient with locomotor disease

- Use physical as well as pharmacological measures to relieve pain
- Encourage movement and muscle strength by using physiotherapy
- Encourage the patient to continue normal life in spite of their disability
- Refer patients early to occupational therapists for aids and appliances
- Encourage patients to keep as mobile as possible
- Be aware that patients may be depressed

The following illustrations highlight key features of common rheumatology conditions: rheumatoid arthritis (**138**); osteoarthritis (**139**); connective tissue disease (SLE) (**140**); and gout (**141**).

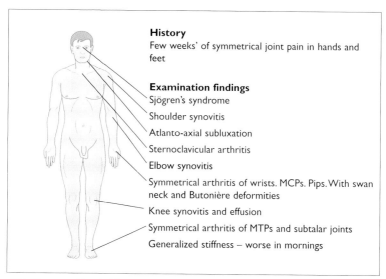

History
Few weeks' of symmetrical joint pain in hands and feet

Examination findings
Sjögren's syndrome

Shoulder synovitis

Atlanto-axial subluxation

Sternoclavicular arthritis

Elbow synovitis

Symmetrical arthritis of wrists. MCPs. Pips. With swan neck and Butonière deformities

Knee synovitis and effusion

Symmetrical arthritis of MTPs and subtalar joints

Generalized stiffness – worse in mornings

138 Rheumatoid arthritis.

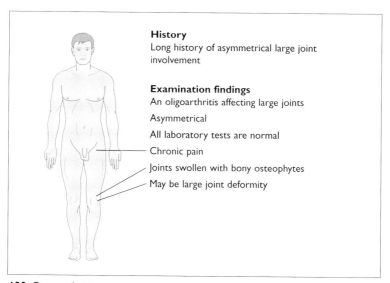

History
Long history of asymmetrical large joint involvement

Examination findings
An oligoarthritis affecting large joints

Asymmetrical

All laboratory tests are normal

Chronic pain

Joints swollen with bony osteophytes

May be large joint deformity

139 Osteoarthritis.

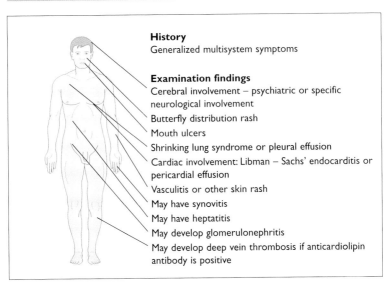

History
Generalized multisystem symptoms

Examination findings
Cerebral involvement – psychiatric or specific neurological involvement
Butterfly distribution rash
Mouth ulcers
Shrinking lung syndrome or pleural effusion
Cardiac involvement: Libman – Sachs' endocarditis or pericardial effusion
Vasculitis or other skin rash
May have synovitis
May have heptatitis
May develop glomerulonephritis
May develop deep vein thrombosis if anticardiolipin antibody is positive

140 Systemic lupus erythematosus.

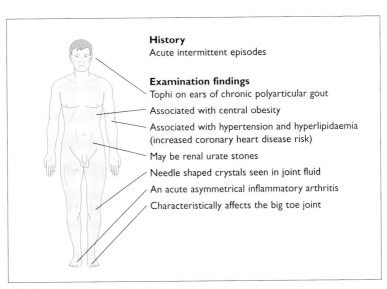

History
Acute intermittent episodes

Examination findings
Tophi on ears of chronic polyarticular gout
Associated with central obesity
Associated with hypertension and hyperlipidaemia (increased coronary heart disease risk)
May be renal urate stones
Needle shaped crystals seen in joint fluid
An acute asymmetrical inflammatory arthritis
Characteristically affects the big toe joint

141 Gout.

6 The nervous system

Most students – and many qualified doctors – find the examination of the central nervous system somewhat daunting. However, such concerns will prove unfounded provided that you remember a basic outline of neuroanatomy and apply some simple neurophysiological principles.

A fully comprehensive clinical examination of the nervous system may take a considerable time: in practice, this is often unfeasible. You should be able with time (and a little experience) to judge the need for a comprehensive examination after taking a careful history of the patient's symptoms. This is an extremely important prelude to the neurological examination, not only because it may help to determine which aspects of the nervous system require most attention, but it also provides useful clues about the patient's mental and intellectual state.

Applied anatomy and physiology

Disorders of the nervous system usually present with a combination of abnormal neurological signs which are often predictable from the history, provided that you are familiar with the anatomy of the nervous system and neuronal pathways.

The motor system

The motor system (**142**) is responsible for the action of muscle groups, i.e. the initiation of voluntary and skilled movements.

- The **lower motor neurone** consists of anterior horn cells, the efferent (those transmitting impulse away from the spinal cord) nerve fibres which pass via the anterior spinal nerve root, and peripheral nerves to the muscles.

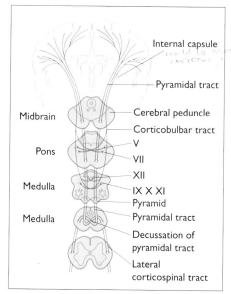

142 The motor (pyramidal) system and location of nuclei for lower cranial nerves.

Labels on figure: Internal capsule, Pyramidal tract, Midbrain, Cerebral peduncle, Corticobulbar tract, V, Pons, VII, XII, Medulla, IX X XI, Pyramid, Medulla, Pyramidal tract, Decussation of pyramidal tract, Lateral corticospinal tract

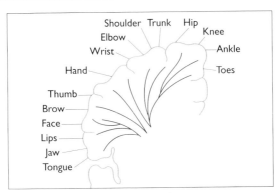

143 Representation of function in the motor cortex (coronal section).

- The **corticospinal (pyramidal) system** consists of the central pathway which directly links the pyramidal cells of the motor cortex with motor neurones in the brainstem and spinal cord (**142**).

- The **motor area** of the cortex is located in the anterior aspect of the central sulcus (pre-central gyrus). Localization of function in the motor cortex with different parts being separately represented is shown in **143**.

- The **corticospinal fibres** descend from the motor cortex into the internal capsule with fibres for the face located anteriorly, and those from the lower limbs posteriorly. They pass through the cerebral peduncles in the mid-brain, the pons, and medulla. In the upper part of the medulla they occupy the pyramids while, in the lower part, the majority of corticospinal fibres decussate with those of the opposite side and pass posteriorly into the spinal cord to form the lateral corticospinal tracts. The corticospinal fibres terminate in the grey matter of the brainstem motor nuclei, or in the anterior horns of the spinal cord. The corticospinal system is concerned with the initiation of voluntary and skilled movements.

- The **extrapyramidal system** consists of those parts of the nervous system, excluding the motor cortex and corticospinal pathways, which are concerned with movement and posture. The system includes the basal ganglia, the subthalmic nuclei, the substantia nigra, and other structures in the brainstem. The connections of these extrapyramidal centres are complicated and include fibres from the cerebral cortex and thalamus. The extrapyramidal system is important in the control of posture and in the initiation of movement.

Co-ordination

The cerebellum acts as a 'control centre' for coordinated movements. The connections of the cerebellum include links with the skin, muscles, ears (both auditory and vestibular), eyes, and viscera. In addition, corticocerebellar pathways provide links with information from the cerebral cortex. The cerebellum uses this information to control the maintenance of postural muscles (particularly those concerned with balance) and to achieve coordination of voluntary movements.

The sensory system

Afferent fibres convey stimuli to the spinal cord. They enter the spinal cord via the posterior root ganglia and the posterior roots. The majority of afferent fibres terminate in the grey matter of the posterior horn, at or near the level at which they enter. The second sensory neurone fibres arise from these cells in the posterior horn (144). Sensations of pain and temperature ascend in the lateral spinothalamic tract, with fibres from the lower part of the body being placed laterally and those from the upper part medially. These fibres cross immediately,

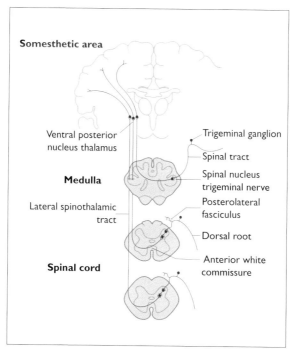

144 The sensory system (pain and temperature).

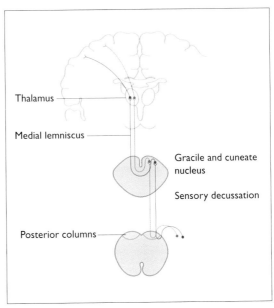

145 The sensory system – proprioception.

or within a few segments, to the opposite lateral and anterior columns of the cord and ascend to the brainstem as the anterior and lateral spinothalamic tracts. Simple touch also follows this route, largely in the anterior spinothalamic tract. The other afferent fibres do not synapse in the grey matter of the posterior horns of the spinal cord, but ascend in the ipsilateral posterior columns (**145**) (joint position sense, size, shape, discrimination, and vibration sense).

At the upper end of the spinal cord the posterior column figures terminate in the gracile and cuneate nuclei. The fibres of the second sensory neurone originate in these nuclei and immediately cross to the opposite side of the medulla in the sensory decussation.

At the level of the medulla, the spinothalamic fibres touch and pass laterally, while the posterior columns enter the medial lemniscus. A lesion at the level of the medulla (or above) will involve all sensory fibres from the opposite half of the body. Higher in the brainstem the two sensory pathways are joined by the second sensory fibres from cranial nerve nuclei (**144**). The fibres of the medial lemniscus and spinothalamic tract synapse in the thalamus. The fibres finally ascend through the internal capsule to the cerebral cortex.

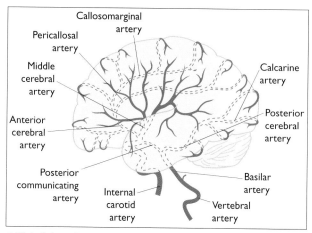

146 Left lateral view of the principal arteries of the cerebrum.

Vascular supply

The brain is supplied by the internal carotid and the vertebral arteries. The blood supply to the brain is illustrated in **146**.

Taking the history

The presenting complaint

If you suspect a disease of the nervous system, then it is essential to take a comprehensive history. Included in this history must be the duration of the symptom, its development, and its subsequent course because this gives you a clue to the underlying diagnosis. Sometimes the nature of the condition makes it difficult to obtain an accurate account from the patient as they may be confused and, in such circumstances, it is important to question a relative, a friend or a witness of any event. For example in multiple sclerosis, the episodes of neurological loss occur in relapses and remissions, with slow progression which may be over several years. The symptoms particularly relevant to the nervous system are shown in **Table 29**.

Table 29. Symptoms of CNS disease
● Headache
● Visual disturbance
● Unconsciousness, faints or fits
● Problems with speech
● Difficulty in performing simple tasks
● Difficulty with walking
● Bowel and urinary disturbances
● Numbness
● Muscle weakness

Headache Headache is a common presentation in neurological disease. It is also very commonly felt by patients with no neurological pathology. In such cases, there may be psychological reasons which should be explored and discussed with the patient.

Determining the site and distribution of the headache may help in diagnosis: pain may be localized to an extracranial structure or may overlie an intracranial tumour. Remember, headache can arise as a result of disease affecting the teeth, sinuses, eyes, ears, and cervical spine (**Table 30**). Migrainous headaches may occur at regular intervals or be confined to particular times, while tension headaches are typically associated with stress. Headache due to raised intracranial pressure is commonly aggravated by movement or sudden changes in posture, and may be worse in the morning.

A headache which has been present for years is unlikely to signify progressive disease, while one present over a period of weeks or months suggests the possibility of an expanding intracranial lesion. The following phrases may be helpful in the assessment of headache:

- 'How long have you had this headache?'
- 'Where do you feel the pain?'
- 'How bad is it?'
- 'At what time of day does it affect you?'
- 'What makes it worse?'

Unconsciousness, fits, or faints Whenever possible, obtain a history and description from someone who knows the patient and/or has witnessed an attack. What the patient remembers may be of great significance. A seizure is characteristically instantaneous, but is sometimes preceded by a premonitory sensation or aura. The fit can be accompanied by tongue biting and incontinence of urine and/or faeces.

- 'Do you remember anything about the attack?'
- 'Did anyone see you fall to the ground?'
- 'How did they describe it?'
- 'Did you hurt yourself or wet yourself?'

Problems with speech Problems associated with speech include difficulties in expression, impairment of comprehension, and indistinct articulation. These problems may not be voiced by the patient – but you should notice the problem during your history taking. It may not be appropriate to continue the history under these circumstances: so you should consider moving directly to the examination.

Difficulty in performing simple tasks Patients will occasionally volunteer problems in accomplishing simple day-to-day tasks – for example, difficulty in doing up buttons.

Difficulty with walking Occasionally, the patient may complain that he/she has experienced some difficulty with walking, and find that he/she 'reels' from side to side.

Bowel and urinary disturbance The development of urinary and/or bowel disturbance is important. Incontinence of urine may occur when higher cerebral functions are impaired as a result of organic disease. It is important to ask about this directly but sensitively, as the patient may be embarrassed, and not volunteer the information.

- 'Have you had any trouble with your waterworks ... ?'
- 'Have you unintentionally messed yourself?'

The retention of urine can be associated with spinal cord or conus medullaris disease, while incontinence of faeces may be a feature of nervous system disease, particularly of the spinal cord.

Table 30. Examples of different types of headache

- Migraine
- Stress
- Brain tumour
- Cervical spondylosis
- Temporal arteritis
- Referred pain – toothache, jaw, sinus, eyes

Checklist for neurological history taking

- Introduce yourself.

- Presenting complaint – enquire about headache, blackouts, etc. Assess the time course of the problem.

- Past medical history – enquire about fits, faints.

- Personal and social history – ask about alcohol and recreational drugs.

- Family and treatment history – ask about a history of epilepsy or neurological disease.

- Systems review (see following box).

LISTEN TO THE ANSWERS !

A scheme for the examination of the nervous system

- Assess speech and mental function.
- Test the cranial nerves.
- Test motor function.
- Test reflexes.
- Test coordination (cerebellar function).
- Test sensory function.
- Examine related structures.

Care of the patient with neurological disease

- Consider positioning of disabled limbs.
- Regular turning and pressure area care.
- Appropriate communication aids in patients with receptive/expressive speech defects.
- Continuity of nursing care for confused patients.
- Prevention of self-harm in patients prone to fits or seizures.

If the patient's presenting complaint does not suggest neurological disease, a series of routine questions will usually suffice to exclude any possibility of disease within the nervous system.

Systems review

Important areas of enquiry are as follows (these questions can be asked as part of the systems review in patient with no symptoms of neurological disease):

- 'Has there been any change in your mood, memory or powers of concentration?'
- 'Have you suffered unduly from headaches?'
- 'Have you ever had any fits, faints, or blackouts?'
- 'Have you noticed any change in your sense of smell, taste, sight, or hearing?'
- 'Have you noticed any difficulty in talking or swallowing?'
- 'Have you experienced any numbness, burning or tingling sensations or pins and needles in the face, limbs, or trunk?'
- 'Have you noticed any weakness in either the arms or legs?'
- 'Have you noticed any unsteadiness or difficulty in walking?'
- 'Have you had any problems in passing urine or opening your bowels?'

Examination of the nervous system

Assessment and diagnosis

If the patient's main complaint appears to be unrelated to disease of the nervous system, and the replies to the screening questions are all negative, the examination of the nervous system may be relatively brief. It should include a short assessment of intellectual function, tests of motor function (including tendon reflex responses), and tests of sensory function.

Examination of the nervous system is complex. A full neurological examination may take you some time. It is quite difficult for the patient to cooperate sometimes, so you may need to take a break, and return later. Also, please remember that good communication and avoidance of jargon is crucial. You are asking the patient to perform tricks that may seem very odd.

- You must ask whether the patient is right- or left-handed – the left hemisphere is dominant in right-handed people, while the reverse is usually true for left-handed people.
- If the speech appears abnormal, try to identify the type of abnormality.
- It is important that you understand the difference between aphasia and dysarthria and are able to distinguish, wherever possible, the different types of aphasia.

Aphasia This is a disturbance of the ability to use language, while dysarthria represents a difficulty in the articulation of the spoken word.

You should test for expressive aphasia by asking the patient to name certain objects – a comb, the teeth of the comb, a watch, the winder of a watch, a glass, the rim of the glass. Ask:

- 'What is this?'
- 'Is this part of it?'

It is not uncommon for a nervous patient to stumble over one or two of the questions, but consistent failure usually signifies an expressive aphasia. Receptive aphasia (difficulty in understanding) is tested by asking the patient to perform simple tasks, for example:

- 'Close your eyes and then scratch your nose with your right hand'.

Patients with a post-sulcus lesion will be unable to follow the instructions.

The recognition and detection of aphasia is extremely important, even when it is a minor deficit, because it reflects disease in localized areas of the dominant hemisphere (in right-handed people, the left). Lesions in the left frontal region predominantly affect articulation and fluency, while lesions in the left parieto-occipital area will impair reading, and left parietal lesions will impair several other associative functions, but particularly writing. An assessment of articulation and fluency combined with reading and writing enables recognition of lesions in front or behind the central sulcus – those in front largely affect expression, and those behind affect largely understanding or reception. Failure of recognition may lead to a mistaken diagnosis of a confusional state, which implies a diffuse rather than localized brain lesion.

Dysarthria Dysarthria may be made more apparent by asking the patient to repeat a sentence such as, 'West Register Street'.

Dysarthria may result from peripheral nerve lesions affecting the muscles used in speech or their neuromuscular junctions, or the nerve supply of these muscles. Alternatively, it may be caused by a disruption of the nerve supply of the structures within the brain which control and regulate the peripheral mechanisms.

Apraxia This is an inability to perform certain motor acts in the absence of motor or sensory paralysis. Damage to the left parietal cortex or disease involving the connections between the two cerebral hemispheres through the corpus callosum, may result in a patient suffering apraxia. An example is the patient who is unable to demonstrate the use of a hammer, but is able independently to pick up the hammer. You should test for apraxia by asking the patient to perform a task, for example:

- 'Show me how you would take your jacket off'.
- 'Show me how you would tie a shoe lace …'

after establishing that there is no receptive aphasia and no impairment of power or coordination ability. The patient does not know how to approach the task.

Assessment of mental state, personality, and intellectual functions

(See Chapter 11 for a detailed assessment of the mental state.)

The appearance of the patient should be noted – is he/she unkempt? What is the state of his/her clothing? Disease of the nervous system may mean that the ability to communicate is less than might be expected from the patient's social status and apparent educational level. However, mental confusion or emotional disturbance will make any assessment difficult. It is important to describe the patient's mental state at the first examination, since future management may depend on an accurate assessment of any changes that have taken place.

Test whether the patient is orientated in time and place by asking the name, age, present location and date:

• 'Can you tell me your name … do you know where you are … what is the date?'

Remember that patients who have been in hospital for some time may have difficulty with the date. Assess whether the patient appears depressed – sad expression, little mobility of facial expression, general slowness of action, agitation and, possibly, spontaneous weeping and less eye contact than you may expect.

High spirits or euphoria, which apparently is out of character with the patient's presenting complaint, may be seen in multiple sclerosis, while general immobility and an expressionless face is commonly seen in Parkinson's disease (**147**).

A change in personality, which is usually reported by a close relative, may be early evidence of disease affecting the brain.

You should discover whether there has been a deterioration in

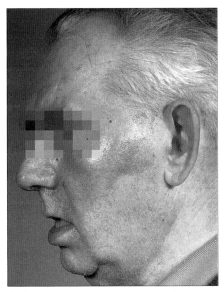

147 Parkinsonian facies. Note the seborrhoea – and lack of expression.

Ten simple questions for a mental test

1	Age	How old are you?
2	Time (hour)	What time is it?
3	Year	What year is it?
4	Name of place	Where are we now?
5	Recognition of two people	Who am I? Who is this person? (nurse)
6	Date of birth	When were you born?
7	Date of World War 2	When did the Second World War start?
8	National leader	Who is our Prime Minister/President/Head of State?
9	Counting backwards	Can you count backwards from 20?
10	Five-minute recall	Can you try to remember this address? (42 East Street)

mental capacity by testing a patient's concentration, memory, and reasoning capacity, to see whether they correspond with an assessment of the patient's level of educational attainment. A test which will help with this evaluation might include ten simple questions (see box above).

Examination of the cranial nerves

It is easier to remember the sequence and the abnormalities if you examine the cranial nerves in sequence from I to XII. The following descriptions outline the important features of each test.

I. Olfactory nerve

You should ask the patient if he/she has noticed any change in sense of smell, and then to identify and distinguish various smells. It is permissible to use objects found by the bedside such as deodorants, perfumes, strongly smelling fruit, and soap. Test each nostril individually and ask the patient to close his/her eyes – unilateral anosmia suggests a nerve lesion, but bilateral anosmia is usually the result of local nasal disease such as a cold. Ask:

● 'Can you smell this?'
● 'Do you know what it is?'

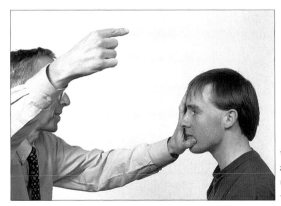

148 Confrontation testing of visual fields; assessment of the upper and lower temporal fields.

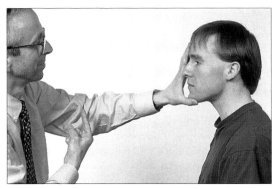

149 Confrontation testing of visual fields; assessment of the upper and lower nasal fields.

II. Optic nerve

Remember to test each eye separately, and that form and detail of vision are best perceived in the central field.

Test the patient's visual acuity (with the patient wearing glasses if necessary) by asking him/her to read small print by near vision, and large print at a distance. Assess the visual fields by the method of 'confrontation' – sit at the same level as the patient, and try to be absolutely opposite him/her, and ask him/her to cover or close one eye. You should cover or close your opposite eye. The patient should then fix the gaze of the other eye on your open eye while you bring into their (and your) vision a pin, or your finger, from the middle of each of the quadrants of the visual field (**148**). The patient is asked to tell you when the advancing object is visible to him/her; compare this with when you first see the object. This is repeated for the upper and lower temporal (outer) fields and the upper and lower nasal (inner) fields (**149**).

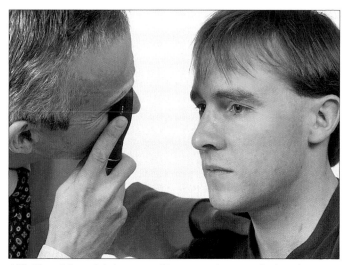

150 Use of the ophthalmoscope. Use your right eye to look in the patient's right eye.

Each eye is tested separately, and then the two together, to check for sensory inattention which may occur in a parietal stroke. You should now repeat the examination using a red pin instead of your finger to outline the central or macular field – a central area of impaired vision (central scotoma) is recognized by an inability to see the red pin compared with your own vision. This is particularly important, as it may be enlarged in conditions such as senile macular degeneration and diabetes, that may affect the macular area.

Use of the ophthalmoscope The optic fundi must be examined with an ophthalmoscope (**150**). Ophthalmoscopy is a difficult part of the examination, and one with which students often have problems. It is made much easier with a cooperative patient. The only way to become adept in ophthalmoscopy is to practice as much as possible. If you do not have perfect vision, you will find it more difficult. Either correct for your refractive problem with the ophthalmoscope lens, or wear glasses or contact lenses.

Always introduce yourself and explain what you are going to do and why. Outline how you will perform the examination and ask if the patient has any

Using the ophthalmoscope

● Correct for refraction. Ask the patient if he/she wears glasses, and take your own visual acuity into account. If he/she and/or you have a significant refractive problem, ask him/her to put glasses on. Use your right eye for the patient's right eye and vice versa, or you will find you are rubbing noses. Make sure you are sitting comfortably and are opposite the patient.

● Put your non-dominant hand on his/her shoulder so that you can gauge how close you are. Ask the patient to focus on a distant object, but warn him/her to keep looking in that direction even if you get in the way.

● Begin by assessing the red reflex. Hold the ophthalmoscope to your own eye and look through it from a distance of about 1 m (3 ft). You should see a red light similar to that seen on the photographs when a flash bulb has gone off.

● Set your ophthalmoscope at the highest negative number on the focus dial. This may be red or black, depending on the instrument you are using. Look through the lens from a distance of just less than 1 m, aiming at the pupil, and gradually bring the ophthalmoscope closer to the patient's eye. You will find that the retina suddenly comes into focus when you are approximately 2–3 cm from the eye. Focus on the anterior structures of the eye before concentrating on the fundus.

● Then focus on the optic disc. This consists of a yellow circle crossed by blood vessels. Note its colour, clarity, and the depth of the physiological cup – swelling with indistinct margins suggests papilloedema; extreme paleness indicates optic atrophy.

● Look at the macula and retinal background structures for any additional abnormalities.

questions. Check the controls on the ophthalmoscope and make sure that the batteries are working. It is a good idea to get into the habit of doing this.

You will need to see several retinal photographs before the technique becomes familiar. Look temporally to see the macula, a reddish blob. It is helpful to describe what you see as you go along. Search the 'background', i.e. not the disc or the macula, for haemorrhages and exudates, and examine the retinal blood vessels, noting their calibre and regularity – arterioles should be about two-thirds the diameters of veins and should be regular in outline.

An example of a normal optic disc and that in diabetes, hypertension, papilloedema, and optic atrophy are shown (151–155).

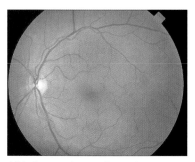

151 A normal optic disc and retina.

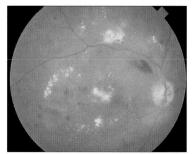

152 A diabetic fundus. Note dot and blot haemorrhages and exudates.

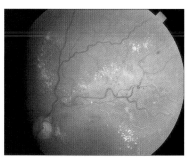

153 A hypertensive fundus. Note the increased tortuosity of the vessels.

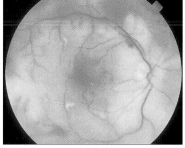

154 Papilloedema. Note the blurring of the disc margins.

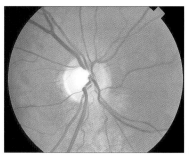

155 Optic atrophy. Note the disc is clear and pale.

III, IV, and VI. Oculomotor, trochlear and abducens nerves (eye movement)

The abducens nerve innervates the lateral rectus and the trochlear innervates the superior oblique muscle. All the other external ocular muscles, the sphincter pupillae (muscle of accommodation), and the levator palpebrae are supplied by the oculomotor nerve. A simple way to remember the muscle innervation is LR_6SO_4 – Remainder 3: lateral rectus = abducens (cranial nerve no. 6), superior oblique = trochlear (cranial nerve no. 4) and the remainder oculomotor (cranial nerve no. 3). The actions of the external muscles are illustrated in **156**. Superior and inferior recti act as elevators and depressors alone when the eye is abducted; the superior and inferior recti act similarly when the eye is in adduction. Normally, movements of the eyes are symmetrical or conjugate – conjugate movements depend on brainstem integration of the IIIrd, IVth and VIth nuclei. Ask the patient to look at your finger and follow its movement with their eyes. Also ask them to tell you if they see double. This suggests a lack of conjugate eye movements, and may occur in nerve palsies. If the patient sees double, it may

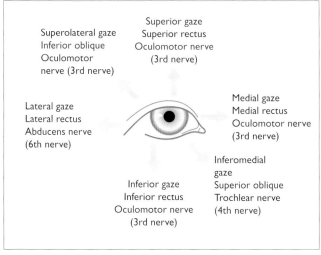

156 The actions of the external ocular muscles.

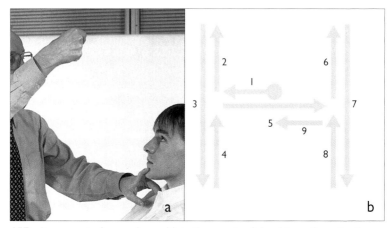

157a Assessment of upward gaze. Note the examiner's hand is on the patient's chin to ensure an appropriate distance between doctor and patient. **157b** The directions to follow when testing eye movement.

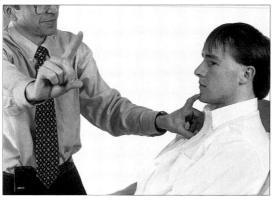

158 Assessment of lateral gaze. Note that, in normal people, looking too far laterally induces nystagmus.

confirm your suspicions. Move your finger to the patient's right, then up and down, then to their left, and then up and down. As in **149**, keep your non-dominant hand on the patient's chin to ensure that you're not too far away – an arm's length is sufficient (**157, 158**). If you move your finger too far laterally, you will see one or two beats of physiological nystagmus – this is normal. Obvious nystagmus in one direction (see below) suggests a cerebellar lesion on that side.

You must observe the size, shape, and equality of the pupils – note whether the pupils are large or small and whether they have an irregular contour. Test their reaction to a bright light. Ask the patient to look across the room, and then shine a bright light into one eye – both pupils should constrict almost immediately (known as a consensual pupil reaction). You should then test for accommodation, asking the patient to look away at a distant object. Then quickly look at your finger which is held close to his/her nose – as the eyes converge to accomplish this, the pupils should become smaller. Look for drooping of the eyelid (ptosis). Ptosis with enophthalmos and a small pupil suggests a Horner's syndrome caused by a cervical sympathetic nerve problem.

Nystagmus This is the term applied to a disturbance of ocular movement characterized by involuntary, conjugate, and often rhythmical oscillations of the eyes. These movements may be horizontal, vertical, or rotary. In any given direction of gaze the speed of movements are usually quicker in one direction than the other. The quicker movement of nystagmus indicates the direction of nystagmus. The patient should be asked to look straight ahead to see whether the eyes remain steady. The patient should then look to the extreme right, and then to the left to see whether any jerking of the eyes are present. This should be followed by the patient looking up and then down to test for vertical nystagmus.

V. Trigeminal nerve

This has motor and sensory functions. You should test sensation to pinprick and touch over the three divisions of the nerve: ophthalmic (the forehead); maxillary (the cheek); and mandibular (the jaw). Remember to keep near the midline as the upper cervical nerve roots may supply the lateral aspects of the face. Compare the size of the masseter and temporalis muscle on each side by palpation while the teeth are clenched. Ask the patient to open his/her mouth: deviation of the jaw to one side suggests weakness of the pterygoids on the same side. Test the jaw jerk by gently tapping your finger placed across the patient's

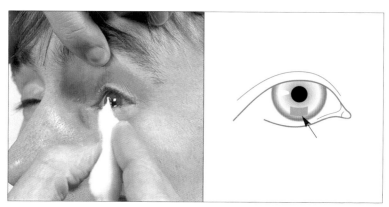

159a Testing for the corneal reflex. **159b** The shaded area over the iris (arrow) shows where the cornea is touched to elicit a corneal reflex.

chin with the patella hammer. Now elicit the corneal reflex – the subject is asked to look straight ahead and the cornea is then lightly touched with a wisp of cotton wool to elicit a blink (**159a**). The precise position is shown in **159b**. You can guarantee to touch the cornea if you are over the iris. If your wisp is outside the shaded area in **159b**, you run the risk of touching the sclera, and getting a false-negative response

VII. Facial nerve

The facial nerve is almost entirely a motor nerve, supplying all the muscles of the scalp and face except the levator palpebrae superioris. The chorda tympani travels with the facial nerve during part of its course, so taste may also be lost on the anterior two-thirds of the tongue when the proximal part of the nerve is damaged.

You should test movements of the face by asking the patient to wrinkle the forehead, screw up the eyes, show the teeth, and whistle. Lower motor neurone lesions of the VIIth nerve or its nucleus produce weakness of the whole side of the face (Bell's palsy), whereas a unilateral lesion of the supranuclear pathways (upper motor neurone) spares the forehead – the patient is able to frown or wrinkle the brow. To test taste, strong solutions such as sugar, salt, or a coffee granule can be applied to the protruding tongue and the patient asked to identify the taste before withdrawing the tongue into the mouth.

VIII. Auditory nerve

Begin an examination of the VIIIth nerve by an assessment of the external auditory meatus with an auriscope. Check that the batteries work before you begin, and that a clean and appropriately sized speculum is attached to the light. It is sensible to examine both ears, starting with the non-affected side.

Hold on to the pinna of the ear and point it gently upwards and backwards, while stabilizing the patient's head with the knuckles of the same hand. Insert the auriscope speculum gently into the external auditory meatus, holding the body of the scope upside down. Look at the external ear and for a foreign body or any sign of inflammation, and then look at the ear drum. It should look pink and shiny. Check for perforation, swelling, redness, or a fluid level behind the drum (seen in secretory otitis media).

You should test the hearing initially by whispering, or by applying a ticking wrist watch to each ear. If there is an impairment, define whether it is due to middle ear disease (conductive deafness) or to a lesion of the nerve (perceptive deafness). Rinne's test is a comparison of the noise heard by a patient from a tuning fork (C256 Hz tuning fork) held close to the ear (air conduction) with the noise heard from a tuning fork placed on the mastoid bone (**160**), (bone conduction). In the normal situation, and in patients with perceptive nerve

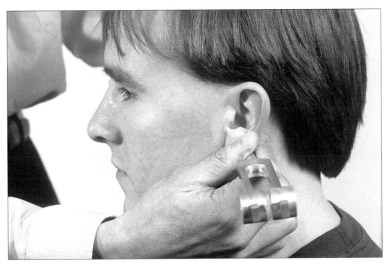

160 In a normal patient, air conduction of sound should be greater than bone conduction (Rinne's test).

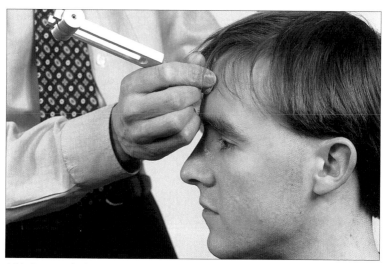

161 A tuning fork in the centre of the forehead is normally heard equally well in both ears.

deafness, air conduction is better than bone conduction, whereas in patients with conductive deafness the reverse is true. Weber's test may also help to distinguish between unilateral conductive and perceptive nerve deafness – a tuning fork placed on the centre of the forehead is normally heard equally well in both ears (**161**). In conductive deafness it is generally heard loudest in the deaf ear, as the sound is transmitted to the nerve through the bone, while in perceptive deafness it is heard loudest in the normal ear.

IX and X. Glossopharyngeal and vagus nerves

The glossopharyngeal nerve is sensory from the posterior third of the tongue and the mucous membrane of the pharynx. It contains taste fibres from the posterior third of the tongue. The glossopharyngeal nerve is very rarely damaged alone. The vagus is motor for the soft palate, pharynx, and larynx. It is also sensory and motor for the respiratory passages, the heart and – through the parasympathetic ganglia – for most of the abdominal viscera. Damage to the vagus is clinically obvious through its palatine and laryngeal branches.

You should note whether the uvula rises in the midline when the patient says 'Aah' – a unilateral palatal palsy causes drooping of the affected side, and on phonation the palate deviates to the opposite side. To test sensation, touch the tonsillar fossa or posterior pharyngeal wall with a spatula – this will provoke a gag reflex in the normal situation.

XI. Accessory nerve

Test the power of the sternomastoid and trapezius muscles by asking the patient to shrug the shoulders while you push down on them (a test of trapezius function), and then to push against your hand placed against their jaw (a test of sternomastoid function) (162).

XII. Hypoglossal nerve

The hypoglossal is purely a motor nerve. Look for wasting or abnormal movements (fasciculation) of the tongue, and then ask the patient to protrude the tongue: a unilateral lesion causes protrusion towards the side of the lesion. The presence of wasting indicates that the lesion is lower motor neurone (nuclear or infranuclear). Tremor of the tongue is common in Parkinson's disease with the tongue either at rest or protruded.

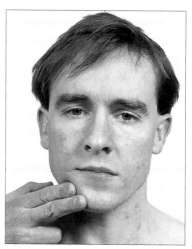

162 Normal sternomastoid function reflects an intact assessory nerve (XI). Note the bulging sternomastoid muscle.

The motor and sensory systems

First, observe the posture and gait of the patient, which may give immediate pointers to nervous system disease – this is done before the patient climbs on to the examination couch.

Romberg's test

● This is a simple test to determine whether an ataxic gait (or a patient's unsteadiness) results from a cerebellar or proprioceptive lesion. The patient is asked to stand with feet together and then to close his/her eyes. Where there is loss of proprioception, the patient immediately loses stability (positive Romberg's test); this is not the case in a cerebellar lesion.

Examination of motor function

You should now observe the patient lying on the examination couch. It is important to observe the patient's overall musculature, including muscle groups which are not visible with the patient lying flat. Wasting of muscles is evident from a reduction in bulk and a 'flabby' appearance. Look also for any involuntary (spontaneous) movements of the limbs, or tremor of the fingers. This may be emphasized by lightly flicking the muscles.

Muscle tone

Muscle tone is a state of tension found in healthy muscles. An increase in tone is called hypertonia, and a decrease hypotonia. Tone is assessed by passively moving the major joints of the arm and legs (elbow, hips, and knees); the elbow is extended and then flexed, the arm is turned in pronation and then supination, the hips and knees are flexed and extended. Hypotonia is easily recognized (it feels 'floppy' and is usually accompanied by profound muscle weakness), while hypertonia may be missed. Spasticity is an initial resistance to attempted stretch of the muscle that increases with applied force until there is a sudden give at a certain tension – the 'clasp-knife' effect. This is caused by a pyramidal, or upper motor neurone lesion such as a stroke in the internal capsule, or a spinal cord lesion in the neck. Rigidity is in contrast a resistance to passive movement that continues unaltered throughout the range of movement, and so has a plastic or 'lead-pipe' quality. Rigidity is classically seen in extrapyramidal lesions and most particularly Parkinson's disease.

Muscle strength

The strength of individual muscle groups in the arms and legs must always be assessed. The innervation of the muscle groups is shown in **Table 31**. Each movement made should be compared with your own strength, or with what you regard as normal power for the patient. It is easiest to make an assessment of power starting from the shoulders, and then working down.

A numerical system for grading muscle power is listed in **Table 32**: this is based on the MRC system of classification.

Table 31. Segmentation and innervation of the muscles to joints

Abduction of shoulders	C5
Adduction of shoulder	C5
Flexion of elbow	C5
Extension of elbow	C7
Flexion of wrist	C6,7,8
Extension of wrist	C6,7
Finger movements	C8, T1
Flexion of hip	L1,2,3
Extension of hip	L5, S1
Adduction of hip	L5, S1
Abduction of hip	L4,5 S1
Flexion of knee	L4,5, S1,2
Extension of knee	L3,4
Dorsiflexion of foot	L4,5
Plantar flexion of foot	S1
Inversion of foot	L4
Eversion of ankle	L5, S1
Dorsiflexion of toes	L5

Table 32. Grading of muscle power

Grade	Description
5	Normal
4	Weak, but can overcome gravity and resistance
3	Very weak, but can overcome gravity
2	Able only to move the limb if supported against gravity
1	A flicker or trace of contraction
0	No movement at all

Assessing muscle power

• To assess deltoid power, ask the patient to push his/her abducted arms up or 'put your wings up', and demonstrate the movement. Then, test his/her power against yours, by trying to overcome him/her (**163**).

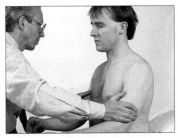

163 Power: abduction of the shoulder (C5).

• Test biceps by asking the patient to hold an arm in the position shown in **164** and say 'pull me towards you'.

• Assessment of triceps power is made by maintaining the previous position and asking the patient to 'push me away' (**164**). Ask the patient to push your hand up (wrist extension) and push it down (wrist flexion) with their hand.

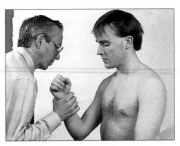

164 Assessment of biceps and triceps. Elbow flexion (C5) and extension (C7).

• Power in the small joints of the hand is tested by asking the patient to 'spread your fingers wide apart' (**165**), and then ask him/her to hold the fingers together while you try to separate them.

• In the leg, test the hip flexors, extensors, adductors, and abductors by asking the patient to push the thighs 'up', 'down', 'outwards', and 'inwards' as shown in **166.**

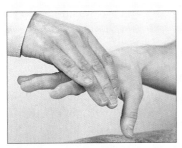

165 Power in the small joints of the hand (C8,T1).

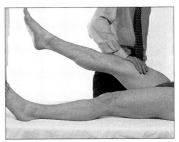

166 Assessment of hip flexion (L1,2,3).

Assessing flexion

● Knee flexion is tested by holding the leg under the flexed knee with one hand and asking the patient to 'pull me towards you', then 'push me away' (**167**).

● For dorsiflexion and plantar flexion of the foot, inversion, and eversion, ask the patient to 'cock your foot up towards your head' (**168**) and 'down', 'out towards me', and 'in'.

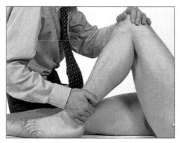

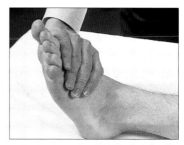

167 Assessment of knee flexion (L4,5 S1,2) and extension (L3,4).

168 Assessment of dorsiflexion of the foot (L4,5).

Tendon reflexes

Testing the reflexes assesses the reflex arc and the supraspinal influences which operate on it. If the tendon of the stretched muscle is gently struck using a reflex hammer, the muscle briefly contracts. This demonstrates the integrity of the afferent and efferent pathways and of the excitability of the anterior horn cells in the spinal segment of the stretched muscle. It is important to become skilled in testing the reflexes: you should always stand on the same side of the bed, elicit the tendon jerks in the same manner, and ensure that the patient is relaxed. Swing the patella hammer gently – and allow it to fall under its own weight. Reflex responses are very variable between individuals in the normal situation – some normally have very brisk responses, whereas the response may be depressed in others. Always 'reinforce' if you cannot elicit a reflex. This is done by asking the patient to grit their teeth or clench their hands together while you try to elicit the reflex again. It is a way of distracting the patient and thus reducing the cortical influence on the reflex response.

System for grading the reflex response

Absent	–
Present only with reinforcement	+/–
Just present	+
Brisk response	++
Exaggerated response	+++

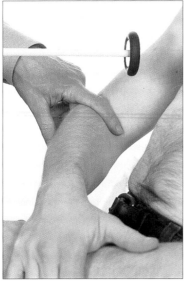

169 The biceps jerk (C5,6).

The reflexes that are commonly tested are the biceps, triceps, supinator, knee, and ankle jerks. Test the biceps by tapping the biceps tendon on the flexor surface of the elbow (**169**), the triceps by tapping the tendon on the extensor surface of the elbow (**170**), and the supinator by tapping the radial surface of the wrist (**171**). In the leg, the reflexes are the knee (**172**), which is elicited by tapping the patella tendon; and the ankle jerk by dorsiflexing the foot to stretch the Achilles tendon, and tapping the tendon (**173**). It is easier to do this by crossing the ankle over the other leg.

Reflexes are reduced or absent in lower motor neurone lesions, and brisk or exaggerated in upper motor neurone lesions.

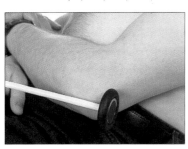

170 The triceps jerk (C7).

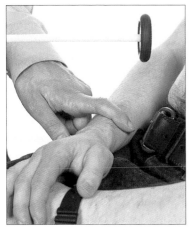

171 The supinator jerk (C5,6).

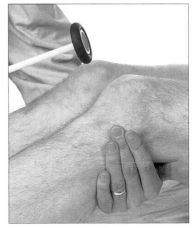

172 The knee jerk (L4,5).

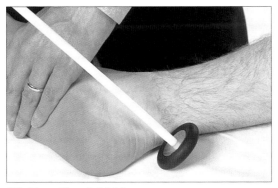

173 The ankle jerk (L5,S1).

Abdominal reflex

A light stroke applied over each of the four quadrants of the abdomen will, in the normal individual, elicit a brisk contraction of the underlying muscles. The upper reflexes are subserved by segments T9–T10 and the lower by T11–T12. Particular attention should be paid to the symmetry of the abdominal reflex response, since its absence on one side may be good evidence of an upper motor neurone lesion.

Plantar response

The plantar response (**174**) is elicited by applying a firm pressure (usually with an orange stick) along the lateral border of the dorsum of the foot, and observing the metatarsophalangeal joint of the great toe. In the normal circumstance the toe flexes (goes down); in pyramidal and corticospinal lesions (upper motor neurone) the great toe shows an extensor response (it goes up, with an associated fanning of the toes). This is denoted as follows: flexor plantar response (↓) down; extensor response up (↑); and an equivocal response up/down (↑↓).

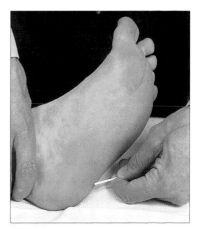

174 The plantar response.

Tests of coordination

These are not worth attempting if the patient has significant weakness:

- The finger-to-nose test: ask the patient to touch the point of his/her nose first with the index finger, and then with the other, and then to touch one of your fingers with the same finger. Ask him/her to repeat this exercise as fast as possible. The patient can keep his/her eyes open while you change the position of your finger. If this is normal, then there is no need to progress to additional tests. If the patient is not fluent, then you should ask him/her to repeat the action of touching his/her nose with the eyes closed: additional difficulty suggests an abnormality of joint position sense (**175**).

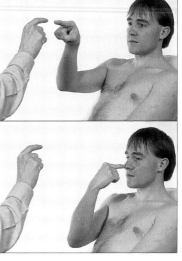

175 The finger-to-nose test.

- Dysdiadochokinesia: this is the term used to characterize an inability to perform rapidly repeated movements. This can be tested by asking the patient to pretend to screw a light bulb into a socket. Another useful test is to ask the patient to perform simple repetitive movements, such as drawing a circle with a finger on the back of one, and then the other, hand. Slow, awkward movements indicate dysdiadochokinesia.
- Heel-to-shin test: to assess lower-limb coordination, ask the patient to slide the heel of one foot in a straight line down the shin of the other leg. In cerebellar ataxia, the heel wavers across the intended target.

Examination of the sensory system

The assessment of sensory function starts with the history because symptoms of sensory dysfunction may sometime precede any objective abnormality on clinical testing. In addition, the patient's symptoms may direct you to a particular area of the body, or the type of sensory function which requires most attention.

The areas and modalities tested will depend upon the type of sensory disturbance suggested by the patient's symptoms and history. However, it is sensible to be thinking whether the pattern fits with a dermatomal distribution, or a peripheral neuropathy. The modalities of sensation are light touch, pain, temperature, vibration, and proprioception. First, test that the patient can feel the stimulus and understands what to do by testing on a part where you know the sensation is normal. Then follow a dermatomal pattern (176). If the sensory

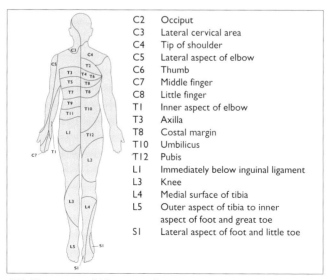

C2	Occiput
C3	Lateral cervical area
C4	Tip of shoulder
C5	Lateral aspect of elbow
C6	Thumb
C7	Middle finger
C8	Little finger
T1	Inner aspect of elbow
T3	Axilla
T8	Costal margin
T10	Umbilicus
T12	Pubis
L1	Immediately below inguinal ligament
L3	Knee
L4	Medial surface of tibia
L5	Outer aspect of tibia to inner aspect of foot and great toe
S1	Lateral aspect of foot and little toe

176 The segmental (dermatomal) innervation.

loss looks as if it is in a glove or stocking distribution, start at the tips of the fingers or toes, and work up until you find a sensory level.

- **Light touch:** this is tested with a wisp of cotton wool applied at a single point with the patient's eyes closed. Do not drag the wool across the skin as this sensation may be transmitted via pain fibres.
- **Pain:** this is best tested using a broken orange stick or a specially designed neuro-tip (which creates a sharp point). A needle point should be avoided because it may easily puncture the skin, and is a potential source of infection.
- **Vibration sense:** this is commonly reduced or absent in elderly patients; nevertheless, it may be valuable in patients suspected of having a peripheral sensory neuropathy. It is best tested using a C128 Hz tuning fork, testing both the lower and upper limbs and the trunk.
- **Proprioception:** joint position sense should be tested with the patient's eyes closed. The system for testing joint position sense in the fingers and toes is illustrated in **177** and **178**. The digit should be separated from any adjacent digits and the joint being tested moved up and/or down. Ask the patient which way the digit is being moved.
- **Temperature:** this is rarely tested as a routine. If it is indicated, then the simplest way is to fill either a blood sample bottle or a metal tube with either ice or warm water. Follow the scheme of looking for first a dermatomal, and then a peripheral neuropathy distribution of loss.
- **Weight, shape, size, and texture:** coins are useful objects for this test. A coin is placed in the palm of the patient's hand with his/her eyes closed, and the patient is then asked to describe it. The weight of different coins can be compared by simultaneously placing different ones in each hand.

Examination of related structures

The neurological examination is incomplete unless related structures are also examined. These include skeletal structures (skull and spine), extracranial blood vessels, and the skin.

- The shape and size of the skull must be observed and the head palpated to look for bony defects or swellings.
- You should examine the spinal curvature and palpate for local tenderness all the way down the spine. Test spinal movements and measure the extent of straight leg raising. Look for limitation of movement of the cervical spine – this is generally the result of cervical spondylosis, but occasionally is the consequence of meningeal irritation.
- Remember not only to palpate the carotid arteries (one at a time), but also to listen over them for bruits. You should also examine the skin for vascular malformations, neuromas, and *café au lait* spots, which may be seen in association with certain neurological diseases.

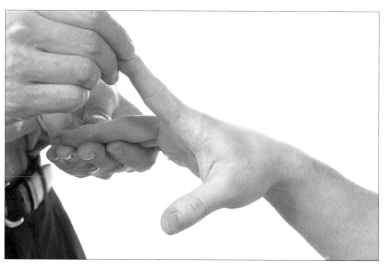

177 The system for testing joint position sense in the fingers.

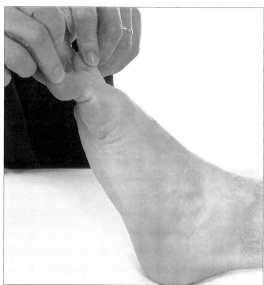

178 The system for testing joint position sense in the toes.

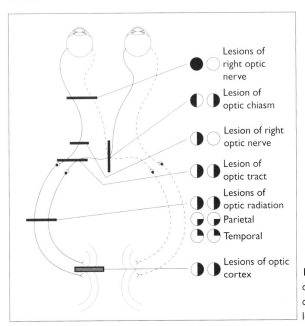

Lesions of right optic nerve

Lesion of optic chiasm

Lesion of right optic nerve

Lesion of optic tract

Lesions of optic radiation

Parietal

Temporal

Lesions of optic cortex

179 Visual field defects caused by optic nerve lesions.

Illustrated physical signs

Physical signs caused by optic nerve lesions (II)

Light from an object on the left side of the body falls on the right half of each retina – the temporal or outer half of each retina is eventually connected to the occipital cortex on the same side, while the nasal or inner half is connected to the occipital cortex on the opposite side by nerve fibres which cross the midline in the optic chiasm (**179**).

A visual field defect may be due to a lesion affecting the eye or optic nerve, optic chiasm, optic tract between chiasm and lateral geniculate bodies, optic radiation, or occipital cortex. A diagrammatic outline of the visual pathways is shown in **179**. Included in the illustration are the common abnormalities which you may encounter, and the anatomical location of the various lesions.

Physical signs caused by defects of the III, IV, VI nerves

- Infranuclear (lower motor neurone) lesions of the IIIrd, IVth, and VIth nerves result in paralysis of individual eye muscles, or groups of muscles. Supranuclear (upper motor neurone) lesions will result in paralysis of conjugate eye movements of the eyes.

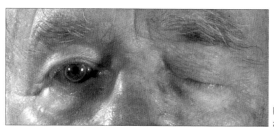

180 A IIIrd nerve palsy. The patient has a complete ptosis.

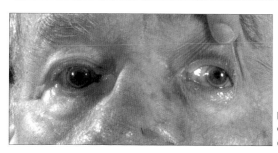

181 A IIIrd nerve palsy. With the eye open, it is deviated down and out.

- In infranuclear lesions of the IIIrd nerve (IIIrd nerve palsy), the eye has a complete ptosis (**180**); when the eye is open it is displaced downwards and outwards (**181**); the pupil is usually dilated and fixed, and there is loss of accommodation. However, the lesion may be only partial, with one or a few of these functions being lost.
- IVth nerve palsy results in an impaired movement with the eyeball being rotated outwards when the subject attempts to look down in the mid-position of gaze.
- In VIth nerve palsy there is an inability to move the eye outwards, and diplopia occurs when this is attempted.

Signs of an infranuclear lesion involving one or more of these three nerves may include:
- Defective movement of the eye.
- The presence of a squint (or strabismus).
- The presence of diplopia.
- Pupillary abnormalities.

Diplopia: detecting weak ocular muscles

● The diplopia may consist of images which are side by side (horizontal diplopia), one above the other (vertical diplopia), or both. Pure horizontal diplopia must be due to weakness of a lateral or medial rectus. Vertical diplopia may be due to weakness of any of the other muscles.

● Separation of the images is maximal when the gaze is turned in the direction of action of the weak muscle, e.g. maximal separation on looking to right indicates weakness of the left medial or right lateral rectus.

● When the gaze is directed so as to cause maximal separation of images, the abnormal image from the lagging eye is displaced further in the direction of the gaze, e.g. if horizontal diplopia is maximal on looking to the right and the image furthest to the right comes from the right eye (tested by covering each eye separately), the right lateral rectus is weak.

Strabismus This is an abnormality of ocular movement such that the visual axes do not meet at the point of fixation (**182**). Paralytic strabismus is due to weakness of one or more of the extra-ocular muscles. The following clinical features are seen in paralytic strabismus:

● Limitation of movement: a prominent feature is impairment of ocular movement in the direction of action of the muscles affected.

● False orientation of the field of vision: erroneous judgment by the patient of the position of the object in that portion of the field of vision towards which the paralysed muscles should normally move the eye. The patient points wide of an object if he/she closes the unaffected eye.

● Diplopia: patients with paralytic strabismus complain of double vision.

The box above contains three rules that may help you detect which of the ocular muscles is weak in a patient with diplopia.

Supranuclear lesions do not produce diplopia, and the ocular axes remain parallel because the supranuclear centres regulate conjugate gaze and do not control individual eye movements. The frontal and occipital cortical ocular motor areas control lateral conjugate gaze to the opposite side, with the result that destructive lesions at these sites cause deviation of the gaze towards the side of the lesion in the brain (but away from any associated weakness in the limbs). The supranuclear centres for vertical gaze are situated in the mid-brain, and lesions at this site produce weakness of vertical conjugate gaze.

The pathways which subserve lateral conjugate gaze pass to the brainstem and decussate below the IIIrd nerve nucleus to reach the pontine centres for lateral

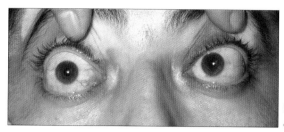

182 Strabismus. Note the lack of conjugate gaze.

conjugate gaze, which are close to the vestibular nuclei and direct the gaze towards the same side. A lesion of the pons producing hemiplegia may therefore be associated with a fixed deviation of the eyes towards the weak limbs.

The fibres from the pontine centre for lateral gaze are distributed to the ipsilateral VIth nerve nucleus, and via the medial longitudinal bundle to the portion of the contralateral IIIrd nerve nucleus innervating the medial rectus. A lesion of the medial longitudinal bundle will therefore produce internuclear ophthalmoplegia, characterized by selective paralysis of the medial rectus on horizontal gaze with monocular nystagmus of the contralateral abducting eye.

Control of pupillary size The size of the pupil is controlled by two divisions of the autonomic nervous system acting mainly in response to the level of illumination and distance of focus. The sphincter muscle makes the pupil smaller (miosis), and is innervated by parasympathetic nerves; the dilator makes the pupil larger (mydriasis), and is innervated by sympathetic nerves.

The parasympathetic fibres control both pupillary constriction and contraction of the ciliary muscle, which produces accommodation, and arise from the Edinger–Westphal nucleus. They travel via the IIIrd nerve to the ciliary ganglion in the orbit: post-ganglionic fibres are distributed via the ciliary nerves.

A lesion of the parasympathetic nerves produces a dilated pupil which is unreactive to light or accommodation. The pupillary response to light depends on the integrity of the afferent pathways, and is lost when the retina or optic nerve are damaged. A unilateral lesion of the retina or optic nerve will result in loss of the pupillary reflex when a light is shone in that eye (direct light reaction), but there will still be a response when the unaffected eye is tested (indirect light reaction).

The sympathetic fibres supplying the eye arise from the eighth cervical and the first two thoracic segments of the spinal cord and pass via the carotid plexus to the orbit. The activity of these fibres is controlled by hypothalamic centres from which central sympathetic pathways pass to the spinal cord.

A lesion of the ocular sympathetic pathways produces a constricted pupil which may become smaller in response to a bright light, but will not dilate normally in response to shade.

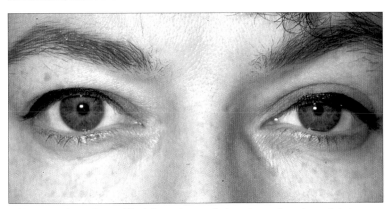

183 Horner's syndrome. The left pupil is small, there is ptosis and enophthalmos.

Horner's syndrome   This is due to paralysis of the cervical sympathetic chain. It consists of slight drooping of the eye (ptosis), pupillary constriction, absence of pupillary dilatation on shading the eye, and absence of sweating on the corresponding half of the face and neck (**183**). Enophthalmos (apparent indrawing of the eye) is often also present. The pupil of a completely blind eye is dilated and fails to react to light, but it does constrict when light is shone into the opposite normal eye.

Nystagmus   This is most commonly due to disorders of the vestibular system, or to lesions involving central pathways concerned with ocular movements, e.g. vestibulocerebellar connections in the brainstem or the medial longitudinal bundle. It may also on occasion result from weakness in the ocular muscles. Nystagmus may be induced by toxic levels of certain drugs, e.g. phenytoin. It may also be congenital in origin, where it shows a pendular quality. A few irregular jerks of the eyes may be seen in full lateral deviation in normal subjects: optokinetic nystagmus may be observed in normal subjects when the eyes are repeatedly fixed on a moving stimulus; an example is seen when a person tries to read an advertisement on a station platform as the train departs.

Physical signs caused by the V nerve (trigeminal)

Lesions of the whole trigeminal nerve lead to loss of sensation in the skin and mucous membrane of the face and nasopharynx, and a reduction in salivary, buccal, and lacrimal secretions. Taste is spared, but lack of oral secretions may result in subjective changes. A characteristic feature is weakness of the muscles of mastication. Pain in the distribution of the ophthalmic division of the trigeminal nerve may be caused by herpes zoster infection.

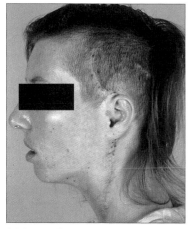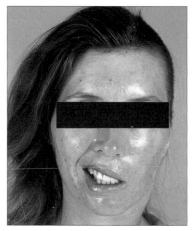

184 and 185 A lower motor neurone facial palsy (VII). Note involvement of the forehead.

Physical signs caused by the VII nerve (facial)

A unilateral lower motor neurone lesion causes weakness of all the muscles of facial expression on the same side of the lesion. There is weakness of frontalis muscle, the eye will not close, and there is a risk of corneal ulceration. The angle of the mouth falls, and dribbling is common from the corner of the mouth. Damage to the facial nerve in the temporal bone (e.g. Bell's palsy, trauma, herpes zoster, middle ear infection) may be associated with undue sensitivity to sounds (hyperacusis), and loss of taste to the anterior two-thirds of the tongue (**184** and **185**).

An upper motor neurone lesion causes weakness of the lower part of the face on the opposite side. Upper facial muscles are spared because of the bilateral cortical innervation of neurones supplying the upper face. Wrinkling of the forehead is normal.

Physical signs caused by the VIII nerve (auditory vestibular)

Tinnitus In the case of the VIII nerve, abnormal auditory sensations may occur. A patient may complain of 'ringing in the ears' (tinnitus). This symptom is common but only rarely due to neurological disease. Hyperacusis is the term used when even slight sounds are heard with painful intensity: this sometimes occurs with paralysis of the stapedius muscle due to a facial palsy. Patients with a sensory-neural deafness due to damage to the cochlea may also complain of a similar problem – an example is Ménière's disease.

Vertigo Patients often complain of giddiness or dizziness. In true vertigo, external objects seem to move around the patient. Vertigo may occur in disease of the vestibular system, e.g. ear, vestibulococlear nerve, brainstem, or temporal lobe.

Physical signs caused by the IX, X, XI, XII nerves (glossopharyngeal, accessory, vagus, hypoglossal)
Bulbar and pseudobulbar palsy Unilateral damage of the pathways from cortex to the lower cranial nerve nuclei (the corticobulbar tracts) may produce transient weakness of the many muscles supplied by these nerves. This results in temporary unilateral weakness of the muscles of the jaw, lower parts of the face, palate, pharynx, larynx, neck, and tongue. There is a rapid recovery even after extensive lesions because the corticobulbar tract on the other side can generally take over function. Bilateral damage (which may follow repeated strokes) results in persistent weakness and spasticity of the muscles supplied by the bulbar nuclei. As a result, there is slurring of speech and dysphagia (difficulty in swallowing), the jaw jerk is abnormally brisk, and movements of the tongue are reduced in amplitude. In addition, there is loss of voluntary control of emotional expression and the patient may laugh or cry without apparent provocation.

A contrasting situation is bilateral lower motor neurone lesions in the same nuclei or cranial nerves which causes a bulbar palsy. In this case, there is wasting and weakness of the jaw, face, palate, larynx, neck, and tongue, with accompanying dysarthria and dysphagia, but a depressed jaw jerk and an absence of emotional lability. In both pseudobulbar and bulbar palsies it is often necessary to feed patients through a fine-bore nasogastric tube – the poor coordination of pharyngeal/laryngeal muscles make these patients liable to aspirate food or liquid.

Abnormalities of the motor system
The ability to walk and to maintain a normal posture of the body when standing are very sensitive tests of the nervous system which are frequently overlooked. These actions require normal sensory, motor, and coordination function: a defect of posture or gait may result from a sensory deficit, muscle weakness, or cerebellar incoordination. Certain abnormalities of gait are distinctive. In paralysis of the dorsiflexors the foot may not clear the ground when walking, resulting in foot drop – the knee has to be raised high as the leg is moved forward and the foot is slapped onto the ground. Proximal leg weakness leads to a

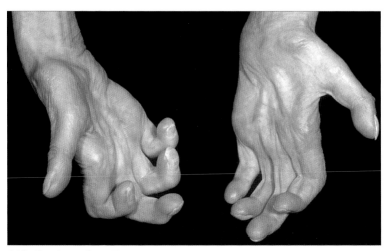

186 Claw hands from T1 involvement in the spine.

curious waddling gait. In a hemiparesis (weakness of arm and leg), the affected arm may not swing and the stiff leg is dragged along the floor. Loss of proprioception in the legs produces a high stepping, broad-based gait with the patient carefully watching the feet and the ground. In cerebellar disease, the rhythmic coordination of the movements which comprise walking are lost, and the patient reels from side to side as if drunk (cerebellar ataxia). Ataxia is made more obvious by asking the patient to walk heel-to-toe along a straight line – cerebellar ataxia, unlike sensory ataxia, cannot be compensated by visual clues.

With regard to the appearance of the muscles, wasting is characteristically seen in lower motor neurone lesions, but may also occur as a result of poor nutrition with weight loss, malignancy, and injury, leading to disuse as a consequence of immobility of a muscle group. In the latter case, strength may be relatively well preserved in relation to the degree of wasting. Occasionally, muscles appear hypertrophied but are weak on testing (pseudohypertrophy): this situation is found in muscular dystrophy, where the muscles are infiltrated by fat and connective tissue.

Muscle weakness may result from primary muscle weakness, a lower motor neurone lesion (motor nerve or anterior horn cell), or a lesion of the upper motor neurone (corticospinal and pyramidal tracts). A lower motor neurone weakness from a T1 lesion causing a claw hand is shown in **186**.

Abnormal reflex responses: involuntary movements

The following more common abnormalities may occasionally be seen:

● *Tics and habit spasms:* these are twitching or jerking movements often associated with anxiety conditions.

● *Myoclonus:* these are sudden, rapid, irregular jerking movements of a group of muscles. They can occur with lesions at many levels in the nervous system, and do not have any localizing value.

● *Tremor:* these are regular or irregular distal movements with an oscillatory character. In thyrotoxicosis, tremors are rapid and fine, but in familial disorders they tend to be of a coarser character (benign essential tremor), while in intention tremor a coarse tremor occurs only with voluntary movement. Intention tremor is best demonstrated by asking the patient to touch your finger and then his or her nose (**175**). A rapid, alternating and rhythmic tremor is present in Parkinson's disease ('pill rolling'), while a flapping tremor (of the outstretched fingers) is seen in association with CO_2 retention and hepatic encephalopathy.

● *Athetosis:* these are writhing movements of a limb. They may be unilateral or generalized; the latter are seen with degenerative disease of the basal ganglia.

● *Chorea:* these are rapid, jerking, and darting movements which may affect the face, tongue and, in particular, distal portions of the arm and leg. Huntington's chorea is an example which occurs in adults and is accompanied by progressive dementia. Senile chorea may be seen in association with widespread cerebral atherosclerosis; chorea is also occasionally seen with SLE and may be induced by certain drugs (e.g. phenothiazines).

● *Tetany:* this is recognizable by a characteristic posture of the hand (*main d'accoucheur*), and is due to hypocalcaemia or profound alkalosis. Inflating a sphygmomanometer cuff above the arterial pressure for 2–3 minutes will produce or augment this sign (Trousseau's sign).

● *Lower motor neurone lesions:* the tendon reflexes are absent with lesions affecting the afferent pathways, the anterior horn cells, or the efferent pathways.

● *Upper motor neurone lesions:* these occur at all levels above the anterior horn cells – exaggerated reflexes (hyperreflexia) follow. It may occur with anxiety or thyrotoxicosis, and is therefore only of pathological significance if it is associated with other signs of upper motor neurone lesion.

Therapeutic and technical skills

Lumbar puncture

This skill may be observed by medical students, but is likely to be performed competently at the Senior House Officer (SHO) level. A lumbar puncture is an invasive procedure which is unpleasant for the patient (187). Remember that they will be anxious about the test, and worried about the results. It should not be performed until the possibility of complications has been minimized. The absolute contraindications to lumbar puncture are conditions associated with a raised intracranial pressure and midline shift. You may want a computed tomography (CT) scan to confirm that there is no midline shift before starting the procedure. It is very important to explain to the patient exactly what is going to happen in order to ensure their cooperation.

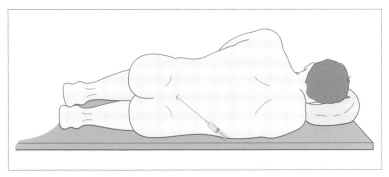

187 Lumbar puncture.

Lumbar puncture procedure

• The correct positioning of the patient is essential to facilitate easy access to the subarachnoid space. It is important to ensure that the patient is comfortable and as relaxed as possible. The patient should be on his/her left side with the back right up against the edge of the bed. The neck is slightly flexed, both legs are flexed and a pillow is positioned between the knees to ensure that the back is vertical.

• Before beginning the procedure, it is well worth checking that all the instruments are functional and fit together correctly. The pack includes a selection of spinal needles and stylets, a manometer, and a collecting tube. It is sensible to check that the stylet fits neatly into the spinal needle, and is flush with the end. The first anatomical landmark is the anterior superior iliac spine. The interspace perpendicularly below this is at L3–L4. The spinal cord ends at L1–L2, so this space or the one above or below are equally acceptable.

• The spinous process just above the interspace is palpated and the inter-space marked in the midline with the fingernail at a position 1 cm below the spinous process. Plain lignocaine (xylocaine) (2%) is used as a local anaesthetic. The subcutaneous tissues are infiltrated first with a 25-gauge (orange) needle. The needle is changed to a 21-gauge (green) one, and the infiltration continued to a deeper level – taking care to aspirate before injecting to check that no blood vessels have been entered.

• It is sensible to allow about 1 minute for the local anaesthetic to work before introducing the spinal needle. The needle is introduced into the infiltrated site at 90° to the patient's back, with the bevel in the sagittal plane and pointing slightly toward the head. The needle is gently advanced through the resistance of the superficial supraspinatous ligament. The ligamentum flavum is reached at a depth of about 5 cm. At this stage, one further push results in entry into the subarachnoid space. When the stylet is withdrawn, a clear colourless liquid drips out.

• Once the fluid is flowing freely, the pressure is measured by connecting the manometer to the end of the needle via a two-way tap. The cerebrospinal fluid (CSF) from the manometer is collected into the first tube. The fluid is then allowed to drip directly into the second, third, and fourth tubes, and the blood sugar tube. The stylet is replaced before removing the needle. When the procedure has been completed, the patient is nursed flat for 24 h. Patients must be strongly reassured if they develop any signs of headache, and given simple analgesia such as paracetamol.

Key laboratory tests

Neurology is anatomically based, so the most important investigations involve imaging. CT and magnetic resonance imaging (MRI) are essential components of neurological assessment – and are a specialist area. The techniques are best performed in conjunction with a neuroradiologist.

The following figures illustrate features of CNS disease: the lateral medullary syndrome (188), cerebral infarction (189), a spinal cord lesion (190), peripheral nerve lesions (191), Parkinson's disease (192), motor neurone disease (193), brainstem stroke (194).

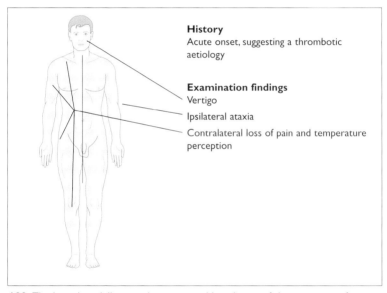

History
Acute onset, suggesting a thrombotic aetiology

Examination findings
Vertigo

Ipsilateral ataxia

Contralateral loss of pain and temperature perception

188 The lateral medullary syndrome, caused by a lesion of the posterior inferior cerebellar artery.

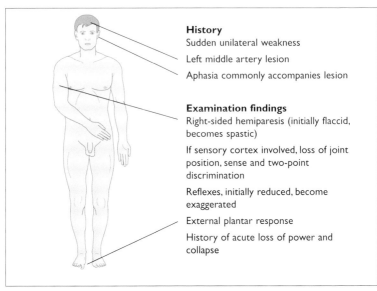

History
Sudden unilateral weakness

Left middle artery lesion

Aphasia commonly accompanies lesion

Examination findings
Right-sided hemiparesis (initially flaccid, becomes spastic)

If sensory cortex involved, loss of joint position, sense and two-point discrimination

Reflexes, initially reduced, become exaggerated

External plantar response

History of acute loss of power and collapse

189 Cerebral infarction.

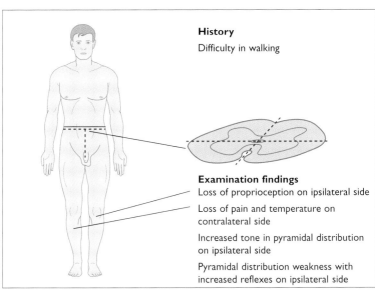

History
Difficulty in walking

Examination findings
Loss of proprioception on ipsilateral side

Loss of pain and temperature on contralateral side

Increased tone in pyramidal distribution on ipsilateral side

Pyramidal distribution weakness with increased reflexes on ipsilateral side

190 A spinal cord lesion.

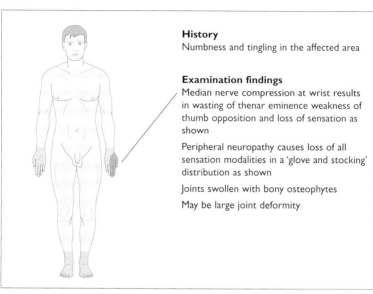

History
Numbness and tingling in the affected area

Examination findings
Median nerve compression at wrist results in wasting of thenar eminence weakness of thumb opposition and loss of sensation as shown

Peripheral neuropathy causes loss of all sensation modalities in a 'glove and stocking' distribution as shown

Joints swollen with bony osteophytes

May be large joint deformity

191 Peripheral nerve lesions.

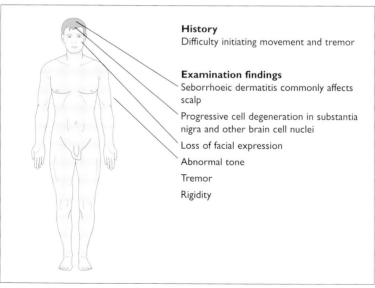

History
Difficulty initiating movement and tremor

Examination findings
Seborrhoeic dermatitis commonly affects scalp

Progressive cell degeneration in substantia nigra and other brain cell nuclei

Loss of facial expression

Abnormal tone

Tremor

Rigidity

192 Parkinson's disease.

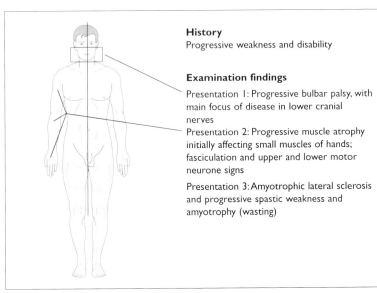

History
Progressive weakness and disability

Examination findings

Presentation 1: Progressive bulbar palsy, with main focus of disease in lower cranial nerves

Presentation 2: Progressive muscle atrophy initially affecting small muscles of hands; fasciculation and upper and lower motor neurone signs

Presentation 3: Amyotrophic lateral sclerosis and progressive spastic weakness and amyotrophy (wasting)

193 Motor neurone disease.

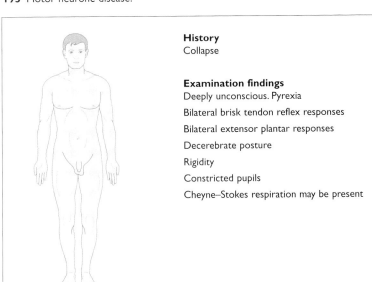

History
Collapse

Examination findings
Deeply unconscious. Pyrexia

Bilateral brisk tendon reflex responses

Bilateral extensor plantar responses

Decerebrate posture

Rigidity

Constricted pupils

Cheyne–Stokes respiration may be present

194 Brainstem stroke.

7 The female reproductive system

Obstetrics and gynaecology

Women's health forms a large part of clinical practice, and includes pregnancy, childbirth, disorders of menstruation, pelvic tumours, incontinence or prolapse, contraception, and fertility. Much of the time the patients are not ill, but the role of healthcare professionals is to identify when something is becoming abnormal, and then to act appropriately. Technological developments are both exciting and diverse, but accurate and sensitive history taking – together with gentle examination – is the cornerstone of good care and will never let you down. To highlight the need for our care, consider the figures for maternal mortality. In a westernized country such as the UK there are 600,000 deliveries a year, and maternal mortality is 8 per 100,000 deliveries. By contrast, in some parts of Africa maternal mortality rises to 1 in 30 deliveries.

There is a wide range of 'normal' in the physiology and anatomy of structures within the pelvis. Additionally, there are variations in function through the lifetime of a normal woman, including puberty, pregnancy, lactation, and the climacteric – each of which can have a profound effect on systemic signs and symptoms. Never be tramlined in your thinking when assessing a gynaecological history. So many systemic diseases can present with alteration in vaginal or uterine function. A good example is recurrent vaginal yeast infections; this is a very common gynaecological problem, but it may be the presenting complaint in women with undiagnosed diabetes mellitus.

Applied anatomy and physiology

The embryological development of the urogenital system is relevant because there are clinical problems which present as a direct consequence of congenital anatomical abnormalities.

The ovaries develop from primitive gonads which are common to genetically male or female embryos. In the presence of XY chromosomes, testes are formed – otherwise ovaries develop. The fallopian tubes, uterus, cervix, and upper vagina develop by fusion of the dual mesonephric systems. The lower vagina is developed from an invagination of the cloacal pit. When the process of fusion is not complete, two uteruses, two cervixes, and a double vagina may be found.

The menstrual cycle

A normal menstrual cycle starts on the first day of a period. Shedding of the endometrium normally lasts 5 days, and is associated with a blood loss of 30 ml. Menstrual bleeding in a normal woman is not stopped by thrombin clotting mechanisms – as a result, a normal period is not associated with blood clotting. After the period ceases, the follicular phase is associated with the development of a graafian follicle, culminating in ovulation on Day 14 of a normal 28-day cycle. The egg is released from a mature follicle, which measures 18–22 mm. Follicles can be clearly seen on ultrasound. Release of the egg can be painful, and has been given the name of 'Mittlesmirtz'. The time from ovulation to start of the next period is always 14 days – the luteal phase – but the length of time from the end of a period to ovulation varies from month to month, and from woman to woman. If the egg has been fertilized, the corpus luteum persists and the next period does not start.

The fine balance of the menstrual cycle is easily influenced. Weight loss for example, reduces hypothalamic function to a point where ovulation stops – few full-time ballet dancers have a regular menstrual cycle.

Assessment and diagnosis of obstetric and gynaecological problems

Taking the history

Many features of the gynaecological history are common both to women who are pregnant and those who are not. The guidelines for general history taking, which were outlined in Chapter 1, still apply. The history must be taken in an unrushed manner, and in an environment which reduces embarrassment as much as possible. An overview of the gynaecological history will be considered first, and then the specific points about pregnant women will be added.

Begin by asking if the patient has children, and how many children she has. Then ask how many pregnancies she has had (see below for details). Establish when the patient's last period was. When you ask, 'When was your last menstrual period (LMP)?', document Day 1 of the last period. Establish when she last had a cervical smear performed, what form of contraception she is using, and her occupation. Ask if the patient has ever had a mammogram and/or a bone density scan.

You may ask several questions to gain an idea about the regularity and usual pattern of the menstrual cycle (see box at top right).

Questions to ask about the menstrual cycle

- 'How old were you when your periods started?'
- 'How have they changed over the years?'
- 'Do they always start on the same day of the month?'
- 'How many days bleeding do you have?'

The presenting complaint

Abnormal periods This is the most frequent problem seen in the gynaecology clinic. This implies a knowledge of what is 'normal', and needless to say there is a huge range of normality. After birth, female babies often have a little vaginal bleeding on Day 2, in response to withdrawal of the oestrogen levels that the baby is exposed to *in utero*. Periods normally start at the age of 11 years (menarche), although quite normally they may start between 9 and 16 years. Menstruation is preceded by breast development (thelarche).

The normal menstrual cycle is 2 to 7 days bleeding every 23 to 34 days. It is not normal to bleed in early pregnancy, and menstruation may or may not restart during lactation. The mean age at which a woman has her last period (menopause) is 51 years, and climacteric symptoms (flushing, sweating, etc.) associated with the menopause last for 5 years in 60% of women. After the cessation of periods for 6 months, there should be no vaginal bleeding. If bleeding occurs after this time, it is very important to investigate thoroughly as 'post-menopausal bleeding' may be the first symptom of pelvic malignancy.

When presenting the history, try to describe the bleeding pattern rather than using terms like menorrhagia or oligomenorrhoea – even though you need an understanding of these terms. Sample questions may be:

- 'When you have a period, do you have to use double protection, such as pads and tampons?'
- 'When you have a period, do you notice clots. How large are they?'

Menorrhagia This is the term to describe heavy periods. The normal blood loss during a period is 30 ml, but when the loss exceeds 80 ml, 90% of women will complain of heavy bleeding. The common 'local' causes are fibroids, endometriosis, and pelvic infection. Typically, the patient will have noticed the passage of blood clots up to 3–4 cm in diameter, and she will have noticed flooding such that she needs to use super tampons in conjunction with other methods of protection. Additionally, the period of bleeding may be excessive. Ask about general problems of bleeding elsewhere in the body, including ease of bruising. There are rare conditions, e.g. von Willebrand's disease, that are associated with heavy periods.

Amenorrhoea There are two types:

- *Primary:* if a woman has never had a period at the age of 16 she has primary amenorrhoea.
- *Secondary:* if menstruation has been established and then stops, the problem is described as secondary amenorrhoea.

The most common cause for secondary amenorrhoea is pregnancy, and this should always be considered as a possible diagnosis. The next most common cause is excessive weight loss, sometimes associated with emotional stress, so ask about changes in body weight, either deliberate or otherwise.

Climacteric symptoms In women with secondary amenorrhoea, ask about the symptoms attributed to falling oestrogen levels at the climacteric. The word menopause means last period. The mean age is 51 years. Premature menopause is when the last period occurs below the age of 40. Hot flushes – particularly on the face and neck – and also 'night sweats' are characteristic. Patients wake at night, fling off the duvet, and go to the window 'while my husband is shivering on the other side of the bed'. Associated with this may be a sensation of dryness in the vagina, short-term memory loss, and other symptoms including epigastric pain/reflux, joint pain, and alteration in body weight.

Dysmenorrhoea When periods have always been associated with pain, and not caused by a specific condition such as endometriosis, the condition is termed primary dysmenorrhoea. In contrast, if painless menstruation has been followed by an increase in pain, and not due to a specific condition, the condition is described as secondary dysmenorrhoea. Pain is described as central in the pelvis, cramp-like with radiation down the top of the thighs, and is often associated with nausea. Ask if the pain starts with the onset of bleeding or whether it precedes it by a few days. The importance of this is that endometriosis is a common cause of secondary dysmenorrhoea and is characterized by several days of premenstrual pain.

Metrorrhagia This is a condition of irregular and unpredictable periods with a menstrual cycle falling outside the 28 (± 5) days. Frequently, irregular periods are the result of systemic hormonal upset. In young women, 'polycystic ovaries' is the most common finding, so ask about excessive hair growth with male distribution, caused by increased circulating androgens.

Intermenstrual bleeding Bleeding in between periods is only normal when it occurs regularly 14 days before the onset of a period, i.e. associated with ovulation. Any other form of bleeding is abnormal, and its cause must be identified.

Post-coital bleeding Bleeding after intercourse occurs as a response to inflammation or tumour on the endocervix, ectocervix, in the vagina, or on the vulva (including the urethra).

Premenstrual symptoms Most women are aware of breast tenderness, fluid retention, and mood swings before a period. Ask about specific problems including depression, tearfulness, psychiatric disturbances, and cyclical headache.

Vaginal discharge The normal vagina is liberally coated by mucus from ducts at the introitus (Bartholin's glands) and columnar epithelium on the endocervix. Discharge increases and becomes thinner at the time of ovulation, and is often absent after the menopause. An alteration in vaginal discharge causing an offensive loss, or a loss which itches, is significant. At this point, don't forget to ask about any infections that the partner may have had.

Pain The normal menstrual cycle may be associated with pain at ovulation on Day 14 of a 28-day cycle, and the first days of a period. This pain should be helped by simple analgesics. Any other pain should be investigated. You must ask about the relationship of pain to the menstrual cycle, bowel function, and urinary function. Ask if the pain is made worse by intercourse (dyspaerunia).

Making generalizations about different types of pain is difficult. As a guideline, pain from ovaries is felt in the iliac fossae. If an ovary undergoes torsion (an ovary with a cyst may twist on the infundibulopelvic ligament), it may pull on the obturator nerve and cause pain down the medial side of the thigh. In addition, torsion of the ovary can distort the ureter, causing pain in the renal area exactly like that of renal colic. However, rupture or bleeding into an ovarian cyst produces sudden-onset pain.

Pain originating in the uterus is felt centrally. Endometritis, for example, gives low suprapubic pain which is aggravated by intercourse. Asking about intercourse is difficult, but questions such as 'Has this problem altered your relationship with your partner?', or 'Can you tell me about it?', will often lead to a discussion if relevant.

Past obstetric history

Every pregnancy is very important. A useful structure to help you think clearly about each pregnancy is to ask about preconception planning, conception (treatments for infertility), the pregnancy itself (first, second, and third trimesters), labour, delivery, the puerperium (including feeding), and plans for subsequent pregnancies.

- Establish how many babies were born after 24 weeks, and ask if they are alive and well – include the names of children. Document the parity; this is the total number of pregnancies that a woman has had, including those that did not produce a live infant, e.g. para 1 + 1 signified one live infant and one miscarriage.
- Ask details of pregnancies that did not go past 24 weeks' gestation. Include details of miscarriages, ectopic pregnancy, and termination of pregnancy. Rather than using the term abortion, it is easier to ask, 'Did you have any pregnancies that you chose to interrupt?' Give the patient time to describe the detail of pregnancy loss, as this is always going to jog painful memories, which may be difficult.

Past medical history

Enquire about previous gynaecological surgery and outpatient investigations, including ultrasound scans, blood tests for hormones, and hysteroscopy (looking into the uterus with a endoscope). Enquire about abdominal surgery, as previous pelvic surgery alters the risks for future laparoscopic surgery.

Breast Ask about the history of benign or malignant breast disease and the treatments used.

Bowel and bladder Enquire about bowel and bladder function. Document the intake of fluids, particularly coffee, tea, cola, and other caffeine-rich products. Ask about accidents in urine control. The loss of urine with sneezing, or even just standing from a chair (stress incontinence), is a highly distressing but common problem for which there are successful treatments. Having to run to the toilet, but not making it in time (urge incontinence), is characteristic of unstable detrusor muscle contractions. Ask also about problems with voiding urine. A large vaginal prolapse for example will often cause an intermittent and slow flow of urine.

Bowel habit is important. Ask about constipation and diarrhoea. Difficulty with evacuating stools may need help with perineal pressure or even digitation with a finger in the anal canal if there is a large posterior vaginal prolapse.

Family history and treatment history

- *Family history:* ask about a family history of osteoporosis and cancers of the breast, colon, or ovary. First-degree relatives with heart disease or thrombosis at a young age may well alter a patient's choice for contraception.
- *Treatment history:* many drugs can affect the menstrual cycle, so make sure all treatments are listed. Also ask about vitamin supplements, homeopathic medicines, and other alternative treatments as these are frequently tried for problems that conventional medicine does not readily help.

Additional history taking in pregnant women

The first visit during a pregnancy is called the 'booking'. Subsequent antenatal visits are short, and are focused on changes since the last antenatal check. Although students see patients in undergraduate examinations during the third trimester, the full history must be taken as if it were the booking visit.

- Ask about a family history of abnormality, including Down syndrome, as well as conditions known to have a link to specific social groups. Sickle cell anaemia is a useful example, but there are many others. Specifically ask about cystic fibrosis, as there is a test available to identify affected babies *in utero*.

- A general discussion about the plans for the pregnancy is important. There are options to discuss about who does most of the antenatal visits, and where the patient would like to deliver. Ask where the patient has been receiving most information, and whether she has attended antenatal classes. Establish which of the antenatal tests have been done, and if the patient knows her results. Particularly important are the screening tests for fetal normality.

- In the third trimester, ask about the symptoms caused by pre-eclampsia. Headaches, visual disturbances, epigastric pain (often more on the right), and irritability are the most dramatic.

Examination of the patient

General

Gynaecological examination includes breasts, abdomen, and pelvis. Also check the height, weight, and blood pressure. It is a terrifying time for women. To help make things easier, the examination room should be warm, and the presence of a chaperone is crucial for male doctors; it helps enormously if support is provided by female doctors.

Examination of the abdomen

The patient should be examined in the supine position after emptying her bladder. After measuring the blood pressure and checking the breasts (see page 222), examine the abdomen. Expose the whole abdomen to just above the symphysis pubis. Observe for scars and distension, and particularly distension arising from the pelvis. Check for splenic and hepatic enlargement with deep inspiration as you would in an examination of the abdomen in any other patient. Check the epigastric area for tenderness and any evidence of mass (significantly enlarged para-aortic lymph nodes would be palpable above the umbilicus). Next, examine the lower abdomen. Start at the umbilicus and with the left hand working down towards the pubic bone, and feel for suprapubic masses. Check for tenderness in both iliac fossae. Examine the groins for lymphadenopathy and hernia (see Chapter 8).

Pelvic examination

Check whether or not you will need to do a cervical smear, and think about whether or not you should take endocervical or high vaginal swabs if infection is suspected. Make sure that you have a light available, a warm Cusco speculum, and the materials for a smear/swab. Remember that this examination is embarrassing and uncomfortable for the patient, so keep her covered with a sheet until you have washed your hands.

● Put on gloves and assemble the warmed Cusco speculum (**195**) (run the speculum under warm water from a tap, but take care that it doesn't get too hot). Roll back the sheets to the level of the upper thigh, and then ask the patient to bend her knees. Many doctors ask patients to put their feet together and flop the legs out to the side, but it may be easier and more natural for the patients to bend

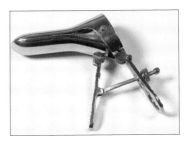

195 A Cusco speculum.

their knees and keep the feet 20 cm apart. Always wear gloves for this examination. Before using the speculum, look closely at the vulval skin, perineal skin, and perianal skin. Identify if there are any scars (including episiotomy), and see if the vulval skin has lost its normal outlines (which is one of the characteristic findings of vulval dystrophy).

● To place the speculum in the vagina, hold it in your dominant hand, while holding the labia apart with your non-dominant hand. Insert the speculum with the handle to the patient's right initially and, as it slides in, rotate the handle anteriorly (**196**). Put the thumb and first finger of your

dominant hand on the posterior lip of the speculum (point A) to push it sufficiently far in to see the cervix when opened. Squeeze the handles of the speculum slowly. If you are unable to see the cervix after slight adjustment, don't struggle. Remove the speculum and check the position of the cervix with a gentle one-finger examination of the vagina, using your dominant hand. To withdraw

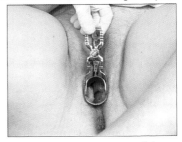

196 A speculum examination of the vagina.

Pelvic examination – continued

the speculum, pull slowly on the posterior blade with your dominant hand, while keeping your non-dominant hand on the handles with gentle pressure so that the blades are slightly open. This ensures that you don't trap any vaginal skin. As you withdraw the speculum, use this opportunity to look at the vagina carefully so as not miss warts, polyps, etc.

● After removing the speculum, stand on the right side of the patient, and perform a bimanual examination (**197**). Lubricated first and second gloved fingers of the right hand are introduced into the vagina. Identify the cervix. Your left hand is placed on the patient's abdomen suprapubically, and gently pushes down towards the pelvis. The size and position of the uterus can be determined by pushing gently on the cervix and feeling the uterus with your left hand. In approximately two-thirds of women the uterus is anteverted, while in one-third of women it is retroverted (**198**). The retroverted uterus is felt by moving the fingers off the cervix in the vagina to the posterior fornix, and pressing gently on the abdomen with the left hand.

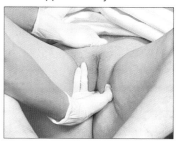

197 Bimanual vaginal examination.

● To feel the right ovary, the fingers of your right hand are moved to the right of the cervix. Pushing cranially, your fingers are now in the top of the vagina next to the cervix (the lateral fornix). Simultaneously move your left hand to the right iliac fossa and sweep your fingers towards the fingers of your right hand as if you are trying to make your finger-tips touch. The ovary will be palpable if it is enlarged. Sometimes it is possible to feel a normal ovary in a slim premenopausal woman.

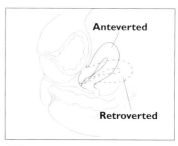

198 Diagram of anteverted and retroverted uterus.

Examining for prolapse

After completing the bimanual examination, the patient can be examined for prolapse. This is not necessary in a young patient who has not had symptoms of 'something coming down'. It is however, necessary for all women who have urinary incontinence, and for those with symptoms of prolapse.

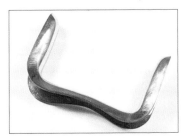

199 Simms speculum, used in examination for vaginal prolapse.

• Ask the patient to lie on her left side and draw her knees up to her abdomen. Ask her to cough, and observe any descent of the vagina walls.

• Using a warmed Simm's speculum (**199**), gently introduce the speculum in the line of the vagina, and apply a little pressure posteriorly to expose the anterior wall.

• Ask the patient to cough again and/or bear down, as if trying to push everything out. Observe at this time the descent of the cervix. In order to do this you need to allow the speculum to gently slide half-way down the vagina (**200**). If you don't allow the speculum to come out with the patient's attempts to push the cervix down, then the speculum itself will hold the cervix in.

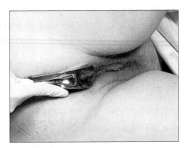

200 Examination for vaginal prolapse.

• Posterior vaginal descent can be observed by replacing the speculum in the vagina and then, with a sponge holder holding the anterior vagina wall away, observe descent of the posterior vagina with pushing.

Rectal examination

It is important to carry out a rectal examination. Assess whether the pudendo anal reflex is intact. As you touch the perianal skin, the external anal tissues contract in a reflex fashion. Also assess the integrity of the resting tone of the anal canal, and the integrity of the external anal sphincter in response to a cough and/or voluntary contraction. Pushing the finger anteriorly into the lower rectum will demonstrate the extent of a rectocele. Do this gently, as rectal examination is extremely uncomfortable in the presence of uterovaginal prolapse.

Neurological examination

Simple neurological assessment includes watching the patient walk and asking if there have been any weaknesses or numbness identified in the lower limbs.

Obstetric examination

Antenatal visits include an assessment of both the mother and an assessment of the baby or babies.

At the booking visit in the first trimester, a normal gynaecological examination is carried out. This need not always include a pelvic examination if an ultrasound assessment is available. Make sure that the uterine size is consistent with the gestation, and do a cervical smear if this has not been done within the previous two years. If there is a history of recurrent miscarriage (more than three consecutive pregnancies lost before 24 weeks' gestation), do vaginal and endocervical swabs to look for infections including bacterial vaginosis or *Chlamydia*. While you are performing the examination, consider two objectives:

- Document baseline values.
- Identify undiagnosed medical or surgical problems, and document the extent of pre-existing illness.

If a problem is identified, consider the management under two headings:

- The effect of the illness on the pregnancy.
- The effect of the pregnancy on the illness.

Assessment at stages of pregnancy

Assessment of the pregnant uterus/baby varies at different stages in pregnancy (**201**). The mother should be semi-recumbent, leaning slightly away from you (never flat on the back, as pressure on the vena cava can cause fainting). Before touching the patient, ask if there are any tender areas, and spend a few moments looking for scars.

● After 24 weeks, look for fetal movement. Establish that the size of the uterus is consistent with the gestation. Using your left hand, feel down from the xiphisternum to the fundus. The medial side and top of your index finger will feel the top of the uterus. Measure the distance from the highest point of the uterus to the top of the symphysis pubis in centimetres, and document this as the fundal height.

● After 28 weeks' gestation, feel for the lie of the baby. This will be longitudinal, oblique, or transverse. There is no easy way to do this, but if you use both hands – predominantly finger-tips – feel once on the left side of the abdomen, and then on the right side. Don't persist if you're not sure, but move on to identify the presenting part, as this may help.

● The presenting part is most frequently cephalic or breech. Other presentations are possible, including shoulder, arm, foot, and cord, but these cannot be felt abdominally. Before doing this part of the examination, ask where the baby has been kicking – a baby that is breech kicks "just where my bladder is", whereas if the baby is cephalic then the movements are felt at the level of the fundus on the side opposite to the baby's back. Put your hands on the abdomen above the symphysis pubis, one each side of the midline with the fingers together, pointing medially. To do this, turn your shoulders so that your back is towards the mother's face. A head shape is hard, whereas a bottom is soft!

● Make sure that the baby is alive. Listen to the fetal heart. You can use a sonicaid to hear the heart from 11 weeks, and a Pinhard stethoscope can be used from 28 weeks. Listen over the baby's anterior shoulder using gentle pressure, but do not hold the fetal stethoscope with your hand as this reduces the volume of the heart sounds. Always feel the mother's pulse at the same time as listening to the baby. This ensures that you have not picked up a maternal tachycardia, thinking that it was the baby. It is sensible to record the fetal heart rate, as abnormalities can be an indication of fetal compromise.

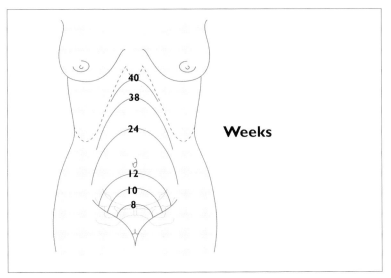

201 The uterus at different stages of pregnancy.

At the subsequent antenatal visits, examination of the mother is limited:

- Check the blood pressure in a semi-recumbant position. The diastolic pressure is taken at the point where the sounds disappear.
- Check for swelling of the fingers, and look for swelling in the lower limbs – gently press laterally on the tibia 8 cm above the medial malleolus for 5 seconds.
- Listen carefully to the mother's concerns and ask about symptoms of pain, tiredness, heartburn, and alterations in the fetal movement patterns. Mothers have a 'sixth sense', and it is a foolish obstetrician who ignores this.

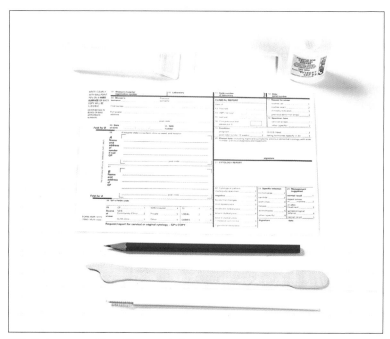

202 Equipment used for taking a cervical smear.

Therapeutic and technical skills

Cervical smear

Explain to your patient why she is having a cervical smear. The ideal time in the menstrual cycle is halfway between periods, but do not do a smear at the time of a period. Tell the patient when and where her result is likely to be available. You will need:

- A warmed Cusco speculum.
- An Ayres spatula.
- A microscope slide and pencil.
- Fixative solution.
- The correct form and a box for transporting the slide.

The necessary equipment is illustrated in **202**.

Taking a cervical smear

● Start by positioning the patient and putting the speculum into the vagina, as described above (page 210).

● Hold the Ayres spatula in your right hand, and the handle of the speculum with the fingers of your left hand. It is useful to secure the speculum by doing up the self-retaining screw, but you will see many experienced gynaecologists who tend to omit this.

● Put the pointed end of the spatula into the cervical os, and rotate it gently through 360° in both directions.

● Remove the spatula and spread the smear on one side of the microscope slide. The result should be a thin film, without blobs of mucus.

● Immediately spray the slide with fixative and label the specimen with the woman's name and hospital number using a pencil.

● Remove the speculum. Be careful to fill in the form completely including the date of the last menstrual period, and information about the use of hormones /IUCD, as this helps the pathologist with interpretation of the slide.

● It is important to warn your patient that she may have some vaginal spotting for 48 hours after the smear has been done, and that this is not a cause for anxiety.

Variations in taking a smear

Occasionally, a smear is taken from women who have had a hysterectomy including removal of the cervix. This technique is called taking a 'vault smear'. The opposite end of the Ayres spatula is used, i.e. the rounded end, but otherwise the technique is the same.

If the cervical os is too tight to accept an Ayres spatula, then a small endocervical brush is used to make sure that an adequate sample is taken.

Table 33. Checklist for a gynaecological history taking

- Previous pregnancies
- Last screening test
  - Cervical smear
  - Mammogram
  - Bone density (if relevant)

- Date of menarche and last menstrual period (LMP)
- Contraception

- Family history
  - Ovarian/breast/colon cancer
  - Heart disease
  - Thrombosis

- Presenting complaint

Table 34. Checklist for history taking from a pregnant patient

FOR EVERY PREGNANCY, STRUCTURE YOUR HISTORY

- Pre-conception
- Conception and treatments for infertility
- First trimester – routine investigations and special tests
- Second trimester
- Third trimester
- Plans for labour
- Labour
- Delivery
- Immediate puerperium (i.e. <24 h) – plans for feeding
- Remaining puerperium (i.e. >24 h – six weeks)
- Plans for future pregnancies

Table 35. Obstetric case presentation

- Name
- Age
- Number of previous children/pregnancies
- Reason for admission/LMP/gestation of this pregnancy
- Past obstetric history
- Past gynaecology history, including menstrual cycle
- Past medical history
- General history where relevant (including drugs/family history)
- Plans for feeding

Table 36. Gynaecological case presentation

- Name
- Age
- Presenting complaint
- LMP
- Date of last screening test
- Contraception
- Detail of presenting complaint
- Past obstetric history
- Past gynaecology history, including menstrual cycle
- Past medical history
- General history where relevant (including drugs/family history)

The following figures illustrate features of gynaecological disease: ectopic pregnancy (203), ovarian carcinoma (204), endometriosis (205), pre-eclampsia (206).

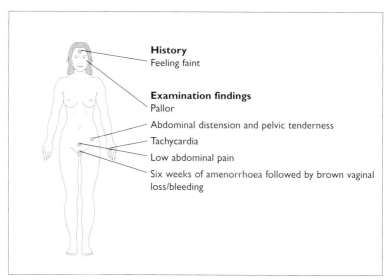

History
Feeling faint

Examination findings
Pallor
Abdominal distension and pelvic tenderness
Tachycardia
Low abdominal pain
Six weeks of amenorrhoea followed by brown vaginal
loss/bleeding

203 Ectopic pregnancy.

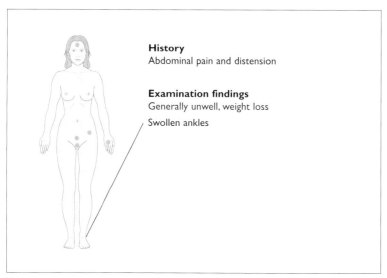

History
Abdominal pain and distension

Examination findings
Generally unwell, weight loss
Swollen ankles

204 Ovarian carcinoma.

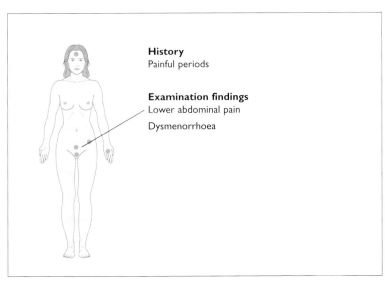

205 Endometriosis.

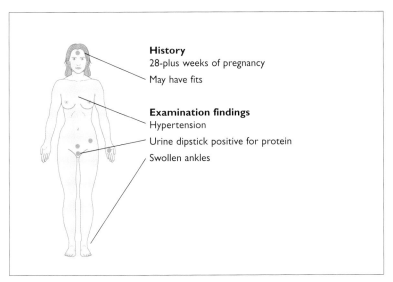

206 Pre-eclampsia.

The breasts

Women usually consult doctors about their breasts because of discomfort, after finding a lump, or more rarely because of nipple discharge. Breast symptoms in men are very much less common, but glandular development of the male breast forming a lump behind the areola (gynaecomastia) and, rarely, carcinoma of the male breast (less than 1% of all breast cancers) may occur.

Discomfort in the breasts is almost invariably benign, though breast carcinomas occasionally present with pain. Breast discomfort chiefly affects women of reproductive age, and may be cyclical – occurring for a week or 10 days before the menstrual period – or non-cyclical. It may be associated with fibrocystic disease of the breast and is hormone-dependent.

Applied anatomy of the breasts and axillae

The breast is a highly developed sweat gland, which has acquired a specialized function. Although there are normally two breasts in humans, accessory breasts may occasionally develop along the 'milk line', which extends from the axillae to the inner surfaces of the thighs. Occasionally, a breast may fail to develop – a condition known as amazia.

The breast has a lobular structure, each glandular lobule draining via a main duct whose opening is on the nipple.

During reproductive life, the breast has a rubbery consistency, and nodules of glandular tissue may be felt within it. After the menopause, it becomes softer and more homogeneous.

Lymphatic drainage from the medial portion of the breast is to internal mammary nodes, which are inaccessible to clinical examination. The central and lateral portions of the breast drain to the axillary lymph nodes, which may be palpable if enlarged due to inflammatory reaction or malignant infiltration.

Involvement of supraclavicular lymph nodes in breast cancer is uncommon but, if it occurs, it does so via the internal mammary or axillary lymphatic channels (207).

The axillary lymph nodes are said to

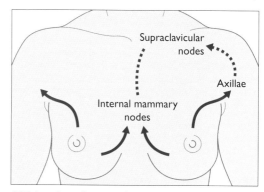

207 Lymphatic drainage of the breast.

constitute five named groups, but the number of nodes present and their distribution are in fact highly variable. Examination of the axilla for nodes needs to be systematic, extending from the lower limit to the apex, and feeling anteriorly and posteriorly as well as medially (208). In breast cancer, the lower axillary nodes are likely to become involved first.

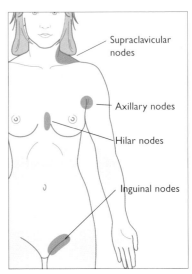

208 Location of nodes.

Assessment and diagnosis of breast disease
Taking the history
Women with breast symptoms, even young women, always wonder whether they might have breast cancer, and some become extremely anxious as a result. Even though the vast majority do not have cancer, the anxiety – and also the embarrassment – associated with breast symptoms should be borne in mind when taking the history. Men with gynaecomastia are also likely to be anxious about their breast development.

The presenting complaint
The presenting symptom – whether pain, lump, or discharge – determines what questions are appropriate when taking the history, as does the patient's age. Sometimes the patient will have more than one of these symptoms.

Breast pain (see Table 41) Severe breast pain of a few days' duration suggests infection (mastitis) which may progress to abscess formation.

Table 41. Causes of breast pain

- Infection
  - Mastitis
  - Breast abscess

- Hormonally mediated pain
  - Mastalgia
  - Cyclic mastalgia

- Rarely
  - Fibroadenosis/cysts
  - Malignancy

The patient may be breast feeding, or may have a history of previous similar episodes. Physical examination will reveal tenderness, induration, heat, and redness of the overlying skin.

More persistent breast pain (mastalgia) may develop at any time during reproductive life, and may also remit. The duration of symptoms, their severity, and whether they are becoming more or less troublesome should be determined – especially whether they are cyclical or persistent. Cyclical mastalgia is always benign, and non-cyclical mastalgia usually so. Is it certain that the pain arises in the breast? Chest wall pain may sometimes be confused with breast pain. Questions asked of the patient might include:

- 'Have you noticed anything which makes the pain more severe?'
- 'How disabling is the pain, and do analgesics ease it?'
- 'Did the pain first begin when you underwent any change in lifestyle, diet, or medication?'
- 'Are you taking the oral contraceptive pill?'

Cyclical mastalgia may be associated with lumpiness of the breasts, or with a dominant lump, which may be an area of fibroadenosis or a cyst. These findings become more common as the menopause approaches.

Breast lumps (see **Table 42**) The differential diagnosis is normally between a fibroadenoma, fibroadenosis, a cyst, and a carcinoma, but rarer conditions should be borne in mind. In cases of fat necrosis, there will be a clear history of a blow to the breast. Skin lesions may masquerade as breast lumps. Sarcomas, cold abscesses, and other lesions are exceedingly rare.

The time the lump has been present is a good starting point.

Table 42. Causes of breast lumps

- Fibroadenoma (breast mouse) (see page 226)
- Fibroadenosis (background of nodularity)
- Cysts (can be aspirated)
- Carcinoma (poorly defined edge, merging into breast tissue)
- Fat necrosis (clear history of trauma)
- Sarcoma (rare)

- 'Does the lump remain a constant size, or is it slowly enlarging?'
- 'Does it fluctuate in size with the menstrual cycle?' (in which case it is likely to be benign).
- 'Is it painful, tender or completely painless?'
- 'Have you had breast lumps before, and if so were they biopsied and what were the findings?'

At this stage, the patient should also be asked about the risk factors for breast cancer (**Table 43**).

It is extremely unusual for patients with breast cancer to have symptoms of distant metastatic spread at presentation. Symptoms which might cause concern would be the recent onset of localized bone pain or shortness of breath.

As the patient may require surgical treatment, suitability for anaesthesia and day-case surgery should be assessed.

Table 43. Risk factors for breast cancer

- Early menarche (before 12 years)
- Late menopause
- Nulliparity
- Not having breast fed
- Breast cancer in a first-degree relative
- A previous (ipsilateral or contralateral) breast cancer

Gynaecomastia in men is usually drug-related (cimetidine, hormones, and drugs affecting hormone metabolism). It is normal in boys in early puberty and occasionally occurs in old age as testosterone levels fall. It may be the presenting feature of a feminizing endocrine tumour, but this is exceedingly rare. The patient should be asked about drug and hormone treatment and the genitalia examined.

Nipple discharge The discharge may be white, yellow, clear, or bloody. Unless bloody, the discharge can be considered to be a glandular secretion, in other words, milk.

Galactorrhoea (abnormal secretion of milk) may persist for some months after the end of lactation, and the obstetric history should be obtained. Galactorrhoea as the presenting symptom of a prolactin-secreting pituitary adenoma is extraordinarily rare, but it is prudent to ask about headaches and visual disturbance, and to check the visual fields. Normally, galactorrhoea is mild, unexplained, and self-limiting. If the patient also has a lump or mastalgia, questioning should be along the lines outlined above.

Bloody discharge normally indicates the presence of an intraduct papilloma, rather than a carcinoma. The patient should be asked if she is sure that the blood is coming from within the breast. Paget's disease of the nipple – a form of carcinoma – presents with a cracked or eroded nipple, which may bleed (**209**).

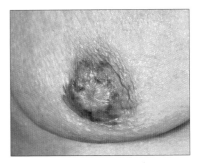

209 Paget's disease of the nipple.

Examination of the patient

Male examiners should insist on a chaperone. The patient should be undressed to the waist. The examination must include both breasts, both axillae, and the supraclavicular fossae.

Inspection of the breasts should begin with the patient sitting facing the examiner, and the arms at the sides. Look for any colour change in the skin, asymmetry of the breasts,

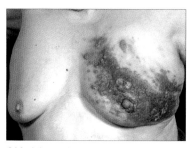

210 Advanced fungating carcinoma of the breast.

and any unusual contour (though the normal right and left breasts are not always of equal size). Look in particular for any dimpling or tethering of the skin, and check that the nipples and areolae are healthy. Local oedema in the skin over a breast carcinoma may produce an appearance likened to the skin of an orange ('*peau d'orange*'), but this is an unusual finding.

Ask the patient to raise her arms above her head and repeat the inspection. Tethering of the skin by an underlying carcinoma is likely to be made more obvious by this manoeuvre.

Care of the patient with breast symptoms

- Appropriate reassurance – most breast symptoms are not related to carcinomas.
- Aspiration of the fluid in a breast cyst may make it disappear – and reassures the patient that it is benign.
- Solid lumps need aspiration cytology.
- Patients aged >35 years need mammography.
- Patients with malignant or equivocal lumps require surgical excision.

A carcinoma of the breast with nipple retraction is shown in **211**.

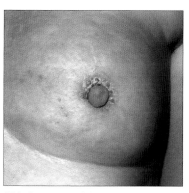

211 Carcinoma of the breast with nipple retraction and *peau d'orange* skin changes.

Palpation of the breasts

Palpation of the breasts is best done with the patient lying on an examination couch. If the breasts are large, it is helpful to ask the patient to place her hand on the side being examined behind her head and to roll slightly to the opposite side, so as to flatten out the breast on the chest wall. It is usual to begin the examination on the asymptomatic side (if any) so as to gain an impression of the texture of the normal breast, which may range from quite smooth to decidedly nodular. Always examine both sides, and ask the patient to point out any areas of tenderness before beginning to palpate (**212**).

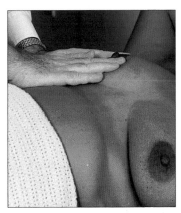

212 Palpation of the breast.

The breasts are palpated by rolling the substance of the breast against the underlying chest wall with the flattened fingers. The entire breast should be examined systematically. A good method is to start below the areola and to work circumferentially, ensuring that all quadrants have been examined. Note that the axillary tail of the breast extends to the anterior border of the axilla and is a common site for breast pathology.

Areas of tenderness are likely to be due to sepsis (look for heat, redness, and induration) or, more commonly, fibroadenosis or cysts. Tenderness is not of undue concern unless there is an associated lump or there are signs of inflammation. Palpation may identify a discrete lump, less distinct lumpiness, or an area of thickening. Thickening and lumpiness may be accepted as normal if they are present in both breasts and there are no other worrying features. A firm lump in a young patient which slips around under the examining fingers is likely to be a fibroadenoma (a 'breast mouse'). Cysts and carcinomas both give rise to firm or hard lumps which move with the breast, but not separately from it. Beware of an underlying rib giving undue prominence to an area of the breast, and simulating a lump.

Cysts may feel relatively smooth and carcinomas more diffuse, but it is difficult to distinguish the two clinically. It is not usually possible to demonstrate the sign of fluctuance in a breast cyst. Large carcinomas may be tethered to the skin or the chest wall. Check that the skin moves freely over the lump, and that the lump does not become fixed when the patient pushes against her hip (which tenses the pectoralis major muscle).

Fine-needle aspiration of breast lumps

Clean the breast skin overlying the lump with alcohol or other suitable antiseptic agent.

Use an empty 10 ml syringe with a 21-gauge needle (green).

Wash your hands and wear gloves.

Keep the lump stable with your non-dominant hand.

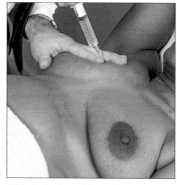

Pass the needle repeatedly through the lump, applying continuous suction to the syringe (**213**). This aspirates a small amount of fluid and some cells into the nozzle of the syringe, which can be spread on a microscope slide, fixed (or air-dried) and sent for cytological examination.

213 Aspiration of breast lump.

8 The male reproductive system

The male external genitalia

The male external genitalia comprize the penis, scrotum, and scrotal contents. Media publicity has heightened awareness among young men of the potentially sinister significance of testicular swellings. Most swellings within the scrotum can be shown convincingly to be benign by clinical examination alone, but special investigations are sometimes necessary. The most common penile condition is phimosis (narrowing of the prepucial orifice), which may be caused by, and predispose to, infection and may cause pain on erection. A wide range of skin disorders may affect the penis, including squamous carcinoma (see below).

Conditions affecting the male genitalia

Painless scrotal swellings
- Hydrocoele
- Epididymal cyst
- Inguinoscrotal hernias
- Lesions of the scrotal skin
- Idiopathic scrotal oedema (young boys)
- Testicular tumours

Scrotal pain
- Testicular torsion
- Torsion of a testicular appendage
- Epididymitis (localized or generalized)
- Orchitis, epididymo-orchitis
- Trauma

Prepucial lesions
- Phimosis
- Prepucial adhesion (normal up to 9 years)
- Paraphimosis
- Balanitis
- Venereal warts, herpes, chancre
- Other skin lesions
- Squamous carcinoma

Other penile conditions
- Hypospadias (minor or major)
- Peyronie's disease
- Urethral discharge (gonorrhoea, NSU)

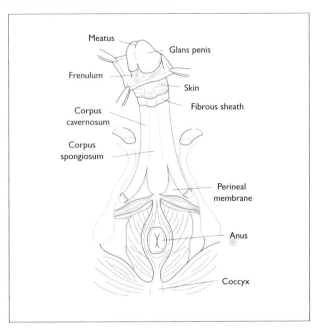

214 Anatomy of male external genitalia.

Applied anatomy and physiology

The **penis** comprises the paired corpora cavernosa and the corpus spongiosum, which surrounds the urethra, and is expanded distally as the glans. Along the shaft of the penis, these structures are contained within a fibrous sheath and covered by freely mobile and very elastic skin, which is prolonged distally as the prepuce or foreskin. The corpora are attached proximally to the inferior pubic rami (**214**).

The **testes** descend from the abdomen through the inguinal canal to reach the scrotum by approximately 38 weeks' gestation. The vas deferens and the testicular vessels thus run through the inguinal canal within the spermatic cord, which takes a covering from each of the layers through which the testicle has passed.

The **cremasteric fascia** is partly muscular, and contraction of this muscle may cause the testicles to be retracted from the scrotum, especially in children. This may lead to a mistaken diagnosis of undescended testicle. So long as the testes can be manipulated to the bottom of the scrotum, they will come to lie there permanently after puberty. During descent, the testicle draws with it a tube of peritoneum, the processus vaginalis, which is normally obliterated during the first 1–2 years of life, except for the portion which covers the testicle itself. Here, it persists as a serous cavity surrounding three-quarters of the testicle (excepting the part which is in contact with the epididymis), known as the tunica vaginalis.

The **epididymis** is applied to the whole of the posterior aspect of the testicle, and is a specialized part of the collecting apparatus, where spermatozoa are matured and stored before travelling up the vas deferens to the seminal vesicles. The epididymis is not normally enclosed within the tunica vaginalis, its posterior surface adhering to the back of the scrotum. This prevents twisting of the testicle on its vascular pedicle.

The **appendix testis**, or hydatid of Morgagni, is probably an embryological remnant of the müllerian duct which gives rise to the fallopian tube in the female. It is a small pedunculated structure which lies on the upper pole of the testis immediately in front of the epididymis. It may undergo torsion, giving rise to acute scrotal pain which may simulate torsion of the testicle itself.

Assessment and diagnosis of disorders

Taking the history

Patients may often feel embarrassed about problems with their genitalia. Thus, questions should be asked sensitively.

The presenting complaint

Painless swellings Painless scrotal swellings in infants may be hernias or hydrocoeles. Hydrocoeles occur when partial obliteration of the processus vaginalis leads to its becoming valvular, so that peritoneal fluid can track down to surround the testicle, but cannot readily return to the abdomen. Intra-abdominal pressure then becomes higher than intrascrotal pressure. The swelling may vary in degree, and may be less marked after a night in bed. Infantile hydrocoele may appear at any time between birth and 18 months of age, and commonly resolves spontaneously before the age of two years, as obliteration of the processus vaginalis progresses to completion. If it persists beyond this age, surgical ligation of the processus is indicated.

The parents of a child with infantile inguinal hernia will report seeing a lump in the groin (occasionally both groins) which comes and goes, and which may extend to the scrotum. The lump does not cause pain, but is more likely to appear when the child is distressed, as crying raises intra-abdominal pressure. It is often impossible to make the hernia appear in the clinic, but the condition may be confidently diagnosed on the basis of the history alone. Inguinal hernia is more common in boys than girls, but in girls it is bilateral in 25% of cases. Femoral hernia is extremely rare in children (less than 1%).

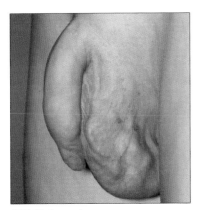

215 Varicocoele.

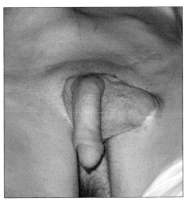

216 Lump in the testicle. The most likely diagnosis is malignancy.

Adult hydrocoeles and epididymal cysts develop over months to years, and present as painless scrotal swellings. The patient is concerned either that the swelling may be sinister, or by the inconvenience it causes. There may be a history of previous ipsilateral groin surgery, but usually there are no predisposing factors. Unlike inguinal hernias, hydrocoeles and epididymal cysts do not change in size from day to day.

Patients with varicocoele (**215**) may complain of a swelling in the upper part of the scrotum (on the left side in 95% of cases). This may be associated with mild aching, though the patients are often asymptomatic. Varicocoele is of concern chiefly because it may be associated with reduced fertility.

A lump in the testicle itself is likely to be malignant (**216**). Unlike most solid malignancies, testicular tumours occur in the young, teratoma having its peak incidence between the ages of 20 and 30 years, and seminoma a decade later. There is usually no associated pain, although there may be mild aching. A history of trauma to the scrotum is not reassuring, as occasionally this may draw attention to a pre-existing lump. It is unusual for there to be symptoms of disseminated malignancy at presentation. An excised testicular carcinoma is shown in **217**.

Scrotal pain Torsion of a testicle gives rise to severe unilateral pain which begins suddenly and usually leads the patient to seek medical attention within hours. There may be a history of similar, milder episodes which have resolved spontaneously. Torsion affects almost exclusively teenage boys. Unilateral scrotal pain may also be due to torsion of a testicular appendage or to trauma, though traumatic pain resolves quickly in all but the most severe cases. In older men, persistent testicular pain is usually due to epididymo-orchitis, when there is associated swelling, tenderness and, possibly, fever. There may have been recent urinary frequency and dysuria, suggestive of urinary tract infection, and the patient may have more longstanding symptoms of frequency, nocturia, poor stream, and terminal dribbling, suggestive of bladder outflow obstruction.

Prepucial lesions   It is normal for the foreskin not to be retractable up to the age of approximately nine years. Below this age, non-retractability, ballooning on micturition, and mild intermittent soreness around the prepucial opening are not indications for circumcision, which should only be recommended if there is a clear history of infection with purulent discharge from beneath the foreskin, combined with evidence of scarring (fibrous phimosis). In adults, inability to retract the foreskin is abnormal, leads to problems with hygiene, commonly interferes with sexual activity, and is an indication for circumcision.

Paraphimosis (**218**) is the term used to describe gross oedema developing distal to a foreskin which has been left retracted. It is uncomfortable, as well as embarrassing, and may progress to ulceration. If the foreskin cannot be reduced after milking the oedema fluid proximally, emergency circumcision may be unavoidable.

All common skin lesions may occur on the penis. In cases of warts or possible syphilitic chancre, a sexual history should be taken. Carcinoma of the penis normally originates in the sulcus between the glans and the foreskin. It is rare in the West and in circumcized men. It may present as a lump or as bloody or offensive discharge from beneath the foreskin. The foreskin is commonly unretractable, but this is more likely to be a cause than a complication of the condition.

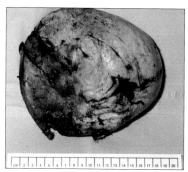

217 Excised testicular carcinoma.

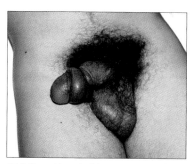

218 Paraphimosis. Note retracted foreskin and a swollen glans.

Other penile lesions Enquiry about penile lesions needs to be done in a sensitive manner, as the patient is often very embarrassed.

Hypospadias is a congenital anomaly in which the urethra opens more proximally than normal. Minor degrees of hypospadias may cause no problems, or may be associated with spraying of urine. Openings on the shaft of the penis, or even on the -scrotum, cause serious difficulties with micturition and sexual function. There is associated chordee (curvature of the penis). Patients with hypospadias commonly have an abnormal 'dorsal' foreskin, but should never be circumcized as the foreskin may be required for use in reconstructive surgery.

Peyronie's disease is a localized fibromatosis affecting the shaft of the penis. It leads to curvature of the penis on erection, and may therefore cause sexual difficulty. There is an association with Dupuytren's contracture, but no causal factors are known.

Urethral discharge is normally associated with **dysuria** and is usually due to chlamydial infection or gonorrhoea. A sexual history should be obtained, and the patient should be referred to a clinic for sexually transmitted diseases.

Examination of the patient

The patient should initially be examined supine, with the abdomen and genitalia fully exposed.

Inspection

This should take in the abdomen (masses, a distended bladder) and the groins (hernias, lymph nodes), as well as the penis and scrotum. Often, the condition of which the patient complains will be immediately recognized. In adults and adolescents, the foreskin should be retracted to check that there is no phimosis and no underlying pathology. If there is a phimosis preventing retraction, then circumcision is warranted.

Palpation

Palpation of the penis may identify areas of fibrosis in the shaft in Peyronie's disease, but is of little value in most conditions. Palpation of the scrotal contents aims to identify the normal structures and the relationship of any abnormality to these. Using both hands, each testicle is picked up in turn. The testicle itself is sensitive, and requires gentle handling. It should have a uniform, rubbery consistency with no discrete lumps or areas of induration which might suggest a tumour. Diffuse enlargement and extreme tenderness of the testicle in an older man suggest orchitis, while a testicle which is very tender, drawn up towards the neck of the scrotum and lying transversely in an adolescent is likely to be torted.

The epididymis should be palpable behind the testicle. It is normally soft, but may be swollen, indurated, and tender in epididymitis. These changes may be localized if mild. A tender nodule at the upper pole of the epididymis is likely to be a twisted testicular appendage.

In patients with hydrocoele, fluid within the tunica vaginalis may make it impossible to feel the testicle itself. A normal epididymis should nonetheless be palpable posteriorly. Epididymal cysts necessarily arise behind the testicle, and may make it difficult to feel the rest of the epididymis, but a normal testicle should be palpable anteriorly. Both conditions may initially be confused with an inguinoscrotal hernia, but may be differentiated from this by palpation of the spermatic cord. It is impossible to 'get above' the swelling produced by an inguinoscrotal hernia, whereas a normal spermatic cord can always be felt between finger and thumb above hydrocoeles and epididymal cysts.

In addition to palpation, scrotal swellings should be examined by transillumination (**219**) using a pen light in a darkened room. Both hydrocoeles and epididymal cysts light up brilliantly when the light is placed behind them. This test proves that the swellings are fluid-filled, and enables them to be differentiated from the adjacent normal testicle. It also differentiates them from hernias (though this should already have been achieved by palpation), except in infants, whose hernias may transilluminate because of their relatively small volume.

In cases of suspected testicular torsion, it may be useful to re-examine

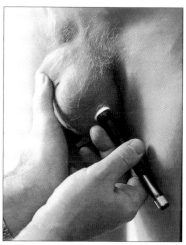

219 Examining a scrotal swelling by transillumination.

the patient when he is standing. This will not only confirm that the affected testicle is drawn up, but may also show that the contralateral one exhibits a transverse lie, suggesting a congenital predisposition.

The inguinal lymph nodes should always be palpated as part of the examination of the male genitalia. It is usual for one of two 'shotty' lymph nodes to be palpable in each groin, but more generalized enlargement may occur in inflammatory conditions and in the rare penile carcinoma. Testicular tumours metastasize to aorto-iliac nodes, not the groins, and the abdomen should be palpated if these are suspected. Examination of the prostate *per rectum* is indicated if the patient has symptoms of bladder outlet obstruction.

Therapeutic and interventional skills
Male bladder catheterization

Bladder catheterization is most frequently required for patients with acute retention of urine. The typical patient is an elderly male who may have a history of prostatic symptoms. Patients requiring an emergency catheterization are likely to be in acute discomfort, so you need to remember this and approach with compassion.

Always introduce yourself and explain what you are going to do and why. Outline how you will perform the procedure, and ask if the patient has any questions. Make sure that you have the patient's verbal consent.

Before beginning any procedure, ensure that all the necessary equipment is there, and check the trolley. A list of the equipment is shown below.

Equipment for male bladder catheterization

- Lignocaine gel.
- Cleaning materials.
- Catheter pack.
- Syringe.
- Sterile catheter.
- Sterile water for balloon.
- Catheter drainage bag.

Bladder catheterization

• Remove your white coat, tuck in your tie, and wash your hands thoroughly at the beginning of the procedure to reduce the risk of infection. Open the catheter pack without touching the inside of the paper. Ask your assistant to open a pair of the correct-sized gloves, and let them fall onto the sterile area, i.e. the inside surface of the catheter pack. Put on your gloves without touching their sterile outside surface.

• Arrange the equipment on the trolley so that it is all accessible, maintaining aseptic technique. Ask your assistant to open a syringe and let it fall onto the sterile area. Ask them to open a 21-gauge needle, and connect it to the syringe. Draw up the exact volume of sterile water to fill the balloon on the catheter (the volume is written on the side of the catheter packaging). Put this down in your sterile area. Ask your assistant for an appropriate catheter. Let this fall onto the sterile area. Ask them to fill the small pot with an appropriate cleaning fluid (normally chlorhexidine).

• Clean the patient's penis using a no-touch technique. This is done by holding the penis via a piece of sterile gauze (in your non-dominant hand). Take a piece of sterile cotton wool or gauze from the catheter pack with a pair of forceps. Dip it into the cleaning fluid and clean the glans of the penis first. Repeat this with a new piece of gauze, starting at the bulb (the cleanest area), and moving away from this, down the shaft of the penis. You may need to retract the foreskin at the beginning of the procedure and replace it at the end of the procedure. Discard the gauze after each cleaning action, and start at the bulb with a new piece. When you are happy that the area is clean, take the sterile towel from the catheter pack and tear a hole in the centre. Pass the penis through this and let it lie on the sterile towel.

• Anaesthetize the area by attaching the nozzle from the catheter pack to the tube of local anaesthetic gel. Lift the penis into an almost vertical position with your non-dominant hand via a piece of gauze as before. Advance the nozzle into the meatus, and squeeze its contents (the local anaesthetic) down the urethra.

• Pick up the catheter from the sterile area. It will be inside a polythene wrapping which is scored close to the tip. Pull off the end of the polythene while holding the catheter through it, but don't touch the catheter tip.

• Dip the catheter tip into some gel (left on gauze by your assistant) and enter the tip into the meatus. Make sure the distal end of the catheter is over the kidney dish from the pack, or you will get wet. Lift the penis, and push the catheter quite firmly until you feel the prostatic bend (you may need to alter the position of the penis at this point). Gently negotiate this bend without using any force and advance the catheter into the bladder. You will know when it is *in situ* because urine will begin to drain.

• Insert your filled syringe into the side-arm of the catheter, and inject the correct amount of sterile water. Then withdraw the catheter until you feel resistance. Attach the draining tube to a catheter bag, making sure not to de-sterilize the join.

• Make the patient comfortable before leaving by making a loop in the catheter and sticking it to the leg. Please remember to replace the foreskin! Make sure the patient is decent before you leave him.

Hernia

A hernia is a weakness in the wall of a body cavity through which the contents of the cavity may protrude. Although the protrusion is usually to the exterior, it may also occur between two adjacent body cavities (diaphragmatic hernia, hiatus hernia), and occasionally between different compartments within the same major cavity ('internal hernia', resulting from intra-abdominal adhesions or a defect in a mesentery).

Hernias most commonly occur at sites of intrinsic weakness, such as the inguinal and femoral canals and the umbilicus. Occasionally, the weakness is due to injury, most commonly surgical (incisional hernia). In adults, the formation and enlargement of abdominal and groin hernias is more likely if the intra-abdominal pressure is abnormally high. This may be the result of obesity or of straining during heavy lifting. Chronic cough, constipation, and chronic retention of urine have also been held to be responsible.

Hernias may cause discomfort and disfigurement, but their clinical importance results chiefly from their propensity to trap loops of intestine. A hernia whose contents cannot be pushed back into the abdomen is termed 'irreducible'. Intestine trapped within a hernia is liable to become obstructed, leading to the clinical picture of intestinal obstruction which comprises colicky abdominal pain, abdominal distension, vomiting, and absolute constipation. Obstructed bowel tends to become oedematous, resulting in a rise in pressure within the hernia. This may be sufficient to cut off the blood supply and bring about infarction of the trapped bowel ('strangulation'). Surgical treatment

Abdominal wall hernias

Abdominal wall hernias (**220**) include:

● Obturator hernia – through the obturator foramen.

● Spigelian hernia – through the lower part of the sheath of the rectus abdominis muscle (which is deficient posteriorly).

● Lumbar hernia – through the inferior lumbar triangle.

● Gluteal hernia – through the greater sciatic notch.

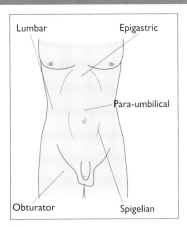

a

following obstruction or strangulation is more difficult and more hazardous than elective surgery, which is why the great majority of hernias should be repaired electively.

Applied anatomy

Diaphragmatic hernia may be a congenital anomaly, presenting in the neonatal period with respiratory distress, or may result from blunt trauma to the trunk later in life. Hiatus hernia, which allows the gastro-oesophageal junction to herniate into the chest, is of concern chiefly because of the reflux oesophagitis which may complicate it. These conditions are not discussed further.

Inguinal hernia This is the most common type of hernia. Two variations occur, which are anatomically distinct but difficult to distinguish clinically. These are known as 'direct' and 'indirect' inguinal hernias.

Failure of the processus vaginalis to obliterate leaves an indirect inguinal hernia sac, which may become evident in infancy, or may remain collapsed until weakening and stretching of muscles and connective tissues in the groin in later life allow it to dilate.

- An **indirect** inguinal hernia passes through the internal (deep) inguinal ring, along the inguinal canal, through the external ring and may reach the scrotum (**221**).
- A **direct** inguinal hernia, by contrast, results from an acquired weakness of the posterior wall of the inguinal canal. It therefore arises medial to the internal inguinal ring, usually remains confined within the canal, and never

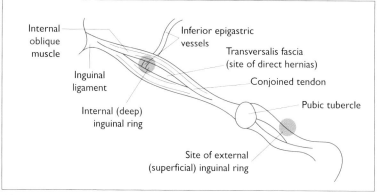

221 The inguinal canal (posterior wall).

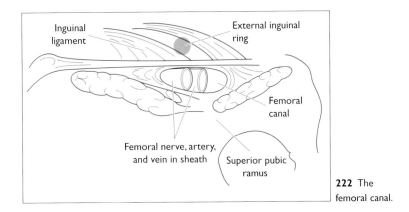

222 The femoral canal.

extends to the scrotum. Direct hernias often have wide necks and are much less likely to strangulate than indirect hernias, whose necks are often narrow. Unfortunately, it is impossible to distinguish a direct hernia from a small indirect hernia clinically.

Femoral hernias These pass through the femoral canal medial to the femoral vessels to present in, or just above, the groin crease (**222**). The femoral canal has tough, unyielding margins around most of its circumference (the inguinal ligament, periosteum overlying the superior pubic ramus). Femoral hernias thus have tight necks and strangulation of small bowel entering them is common.

Umbilical/para-umbilical, epigastric, and other ventral hernias

- An **umbilical hernia** is a congenital abnormality resulting from failure of the umbilicus to obliterate in early life. Umbilical hernias never strangulate, and most close spontaneously by the age of 3–6 years. The main cause for concern is parental anxiety over the peculiar appearance, and surgical closure after the age of three years may be justified for this reason.
- **Para-umbilical hernias** are acquired defects immediately superior to the umbilicus in obese adults. These hernias are liable to enlarge with the passage of time, and not infrequently strangulate. Although the patients are often elderly and unfit, elective repair should be undertaken unless the contraindications are very strong.
- **Epigastric hernias** may present in childhood as a small tender lump in the mid-line. Occasionally, the hernia cannot be felt at all and the child complains only of epigastric pain, which is commonly made worse by exercise.

Epigastric hernias are small congenital defects in the linea alba through which preperitoneal fat protrudes. Surgical repair is justified by the symptoms.

- Adults may also develop **mid-line abdominal hernias,** though often the bulge is due to separation of the rectus abdominis muscles and attenuation of the linea alba ('divarication of the recti'). A mid-line hernia with a distinct neck which has fibrous margins should be repaired, as these hernias tend to enlarge, may become massive, and may strangulate. Divarication of the recti is a harmless condition, however, and the results of surgical treatment are often poor.

- **Incisional hernias** are most common following long mid-line abdominal incisions, though they may occur at other sites. Postoperative wound infection and obesity are the main predisposing causes (along with poor surgical technique). Herniation is due to separation or attenuation of the musculofascial layer. Incisional hernias tend to enlarge, sometimes to massive proportions, and may strangulate. Early surgical repair should therefore be undertaken.

Assessment and diagnosis of external abdominal hernias

Taking the history
Presenting complaint
A patient with a hernia will usually have a painful lump which appears or enlarges with coughing. He will normally complain of a bulge. There may be associated discomfort, especially on straining. Rarely, with irreducible hernias, there may be disturbance of bowel function. Patients who have developed intestinal obstruction are likely to present as emergencies complaining of some or all of the symptoms of this condition, namely colicky abdominal pain, abdominal distension, vomiting, and absolute constipation (passage of neither faeces nor flatus).

Past medical history
As the patient may well require surgical treatment, enquiry should be made about concurrent and previous illnesses and current drug treatment, all of which affect perioperative risk and anaesthetic technique. Some patients will have recurrent hernias, having undergone a previous repair at the same site. This will make the surgery more difficult and may rule out repair as a day case.

Examination for groin hernias

The cardiovascular and respiratory systems should be examined to detect conditions which may affect suitability for anaesthesia.

If the hernia is evident while the patient is lying, examine it first in this position.

● Look at its site and size and, in acute cases, for any inflammation of the overlying skin which would suggest the presence of strangulated bowel within. It is not, however, possible to determine whether a groin hernia is inguinal or femoral by inspection.

● Palpate the hernia gently to assess tenderness, and try gently to reduce it. Locate the pubic tubercle and determine the relationship of the hernia to this (**214**). Femoral hernias emerge below the inguinal ligament, and therefore below and lateral to the pubic tubercle. Inguinal hernias originate in the inguinal canal, above the inguinal ligament and pubic tubercle and, if they extend to or beyond the neck of the scrotum, they pass above and then medial to the tubercle. Note that the inguinal ligament, which runs from the anterior superior iliac spine to the pubic tubercle, lies approximately 3 cm above the groin crease. Femoral hernias therefore present above the groin crease, though below the inguinal ligament.

Despite statements to the contrary in several textbooks, it is not possible to distinguish a direct from an indirect inguinal hernia by clinical examination, unless the hernia extends to the scrotum (when it must be indirect).

Sometimes the hernia is not apparent when the patient is lying down. In this case, he or she should be asked to stand, and if necessary to cough, in order to push it out. This manoeuvre should also be used to check that there is not a small hernia on the opposite side, which may not have been noticed by the patient (though a 'cough impulse' in the asymptomatic groin may be a normal finding and is not, on its own, sufficient grounds for diagnosing a hernia). It is difficult to palpate the pubic tubercle with the patient standing, however, and once the hernia has been demonstrated the patient should be asked to lie down again in order to determine its relationship to the tubercle. In men, examination of a groin hernia finishes with an examination of the external genitalia.

Occasionally in adults – and usually in children – it may not be possible to demonstrate the hernia in the clinic, however much the patient coughs and strains. However, a history of a lump in the groin which appears on standing and straining and disappears on lying is diagnostic of a hernia, and justifies surgical treatment. The precise anatomy can be determined intraoperatively.

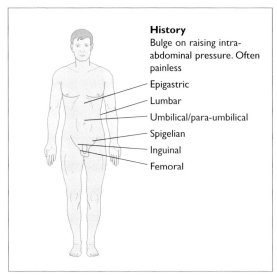

History
Bulge on raising intra-abdominal pressure. Often painless

Epigastric

Lumbar

Umbilical/para-umbilical

Spigelian

Inguinal

Femoral

223 Assessment of external abdominal hernias.

Personal and social history

Occupation should be enquired about, though patients should be able to return to all but the heaviest jobs following hernia repair. As most hernias can be repaired as day cases, the availability of a relative or friend who can escort the patient home, and accommodation which does not require the patient to climb numerous flights of stairs, are prerequisites. The fact that the patient is retired does not weaken the indications for surgery, as strangulation may occur at any age and is especially dangerous in the elderly.

Other abdominal hernias (223)

Once again, the cardiovascular and respiratory systems should be examined. Abdominal examination begins with inspection.

- Look to see whether the hernia is apparent with the patient supine, and for surgical scars which may suggest an underlying incisional hernia. If the hernia is not apparent, ask the patient to raise their head and shoulders off the pillow. This tenses the muscles, raises intra-abdominal pressure, and usually makes the hernia protrude. If this fails, inspect the abdomen with the patient standing.
- Palpate the hernia gently to detect tenderness, and then try gently to reduce it. Feel for the fibrous margins of the defect, which may barely admit a finger-tip in infantile umbilical hernia, but which may be very wide in incisional and some other ventral hernias. A general abdominal examination should then be completed.

Illustrated physical signs

The two photographs illustrate hernial defects: large bilateral inguinal herniae (224); an incisional hernia (225).

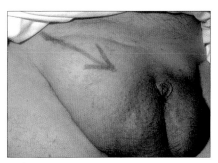

224 Bilateral inguinal herniae.

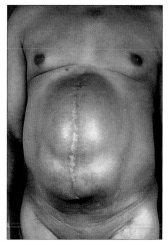

225 Incisional hernia.

Care of the patient with a hernia

- Adult patients should be advised to have all hernias repaired except wide necked direct inguinal hernia.
- A truss may relieve pain – but does not prevent strangulation.
- Most uncomplicated hernias can be repaired as a day case.
- Irreducibility does not always suggest obstruction.
- An obstructed hernia is a surgical emergency.

9 The endocrine system

Disorders of endocrine function, which are not uncommon in clinical practice, tend to present with non-specific symptoms. As a consequence, the unwary clinician may overlook the possibility that either a deficiency (hypo-function) or excess (hyper-function) of a particular hormone or hormones may be the underlying problem. This emphasizes the importance of always taking a comprehensive history and applying the clues provided when performing the general examination. Remember that hormonal deficiency may affect the function of several different organs.

Applied anatomy and physiology

The hypothalamus contains many vital centres for functions such as appetite, thirst, thermal regulation, and sleep/waking. It also plays a role in circadian rhythm, the menstrual cycle, stress, and mood. Releasing factors produced in the hypothalamus reach the pituitary via the portal system and run down the pituitary stalk. These releasing factors stimulate or inhibit the production of hormones by the anterior pituitary which, in turn, stimulates or inhibits the peripheral glands or tissues.

The posterior pituitary acts as a storage organ for antidiuretic hormone (arginine vasopressin) and oxytocin, which are synthesized in the supraoptic and paraventricular nuclei in the anterior hypothalamus, and pass to the posterior pituitary via an axon within the pituitary stalk. Endocrine abnormalities result from either a primary or secondary abnormality, causing either excess or deficiency of pituitary hormone. Examples of the former are hyper- and hypothyroidism. An example of the latter is the production of excessive adrenocorticotrophic hormone (ACTH) in Cushing's (pituitary-dependent) disease. Partial degrees of excess or deficiency may be difficult to detect unless a clinician is wary of the likely presenting features. In contrast, absolute deficiency or marked excess usually present with characteristics symptoms and signs.

The thyroid gland

Disease of the thyroid gland most commonly presents with swelling, which may affect the whole gland (a goitre), or may be localized within it. Less often, the patient may present with signs of over- or under-secretion of thyroid hormones (with or without swelling). Pain arising in the thyroid gland is rare.

Clinical assessment of thyroid disease involves an assessment of the gland itself, related structures in the neck and 'thyroid status' (the quantity of hormone being produced). It is easy to neglect one or more of these aspects, and a methodical and practised approach is required in order to ensure that the assessment is thorough.

Applied anatomy and physiology

The thyroid gland consists of two lobes, joined by the isthmus just below the cricoid cartilage. The gland develops as a downgrowth (the thyroglossal duct) from the primitive pharynx.

This section will focus on the clinical pointers, and indicate the possibility of an underlying endocrine abnormality. Readers should refer to a specific textbook for more detailed information about the causes of the various hormonal deficiencies and excesses.

Assessment and diagnosis of endocrine disease

A high index of suspicion is necessary for the diagnosis of endocrine disease, as a hormonal problem may affect any of the body systems.

Taking the history

You need to ensure that you cover areas of general health. Endocrine dysfunction may often be manifested by non-specific symptoms that will be missed unless a full review of systems is completed. Particular enquiries that should be made are outlined in the following section.

The presenting complaint

Body weight Hypothyroidism is commonly associated with weight gain; Cushing's syndrome may be accompanied by weight gain, particularly in the upper body ('truncal obesity'). Hypoadrenalism or hyperthyroidism are associated with weight loss. The patient might be asked:
- 'How has your weight been recently?'

Appetite An increase in appetite is a frequent association with hyperthyroidism, and less commonly with Cushing's syndrome. In hyperthyroidism, the increased appetite is frequently associated with weight loss. By contrast, hypoadrenalism frequently presents with anorexia and malaise.

Fatigue Many patients with diabetes mellitus will confess to a feeling of profound fatigue for many months before the diagnosis, as a result of unsuspected hyperglycaemia. Similarly, fatigue may be a feature of Cushing's syndrome, hypoadrenalism, hypothyroidism, and hypercalcaemia.

Thirst Increased thirst is a common presenting feature of diabetes mellitus, but it may also be seen in hypercalcaemia and diabetes insipidus. In the latter condition, the thirst is so severe that patients frequently report that they drink a jug of water during the night.

Frequency of micturition Diabetes mellitus and diabetes insipidus are both accompanied by an increased frequency of urination, and the passage of moderate to large volumes of urine. Both conditions are associated with both day-time and nocturnal frequency, although in diabetes insipidus patients tend to pass greater volumes of pale (diluted) urine. Prostatism is usually differentiated by its association with a complaint of urinary hesitancy and the passage of small volumes of urine. Polyuria is also seen in patients who are hypercalcaemic. Remember that patients with Cushing's syndrome may also develop diabetes mellitus.

Disturbances of bowel function Patients with hypothyroidism may complain of constipation, while diarrhoea may result in the referral of a hyperthyroid patient to a gastroenterologist. A patient with an elevated plasma calcium level may present with abdominal pain, either as a consequence of constipation or due to pancreatitis (a sequel to hypercalcaemia).

Sexual function An early symptom that is suggestive of pituitary dysfunction in women is the development of altered menstrual function and, ultimately, amenorrhoea. A delay in menarche (onset of periods) may be the presenting complaint in a girl who is prepubertal. In men, hypogonadism presents with loss of sexual drive or libido, and failure to achieve or sustain an erection.

Headache Although this is a non-specific symptom – and one which accompanies many disease processes – it should be regarded with seriousness in a patient who appears to have an endocrine dysfunction. An expanding pituitary tumour or hypothalamic mass may lead to an endocrine dysfunction, and/or may cause pressure symptoms which present as a headache.

Alteration in growth Hypopituitarism and growth hormone deficiency in children may present with short stature. In contrast, excess of growth hormone causes gigantism in children and acromegaly in adults (after fusion of epiphyses). The latter condition may lead to patients complaining of increase in hand size or, more commonly, shoe size.

Neck lump Patients with thyroid disease may present with a lump in the neck, although this is usually painless.

Examination of the patient
Specific points on examination
An examination of the endocrine system is performed as part of a general physical examination, at which time a large number of endocrine signs are noticed. The thyroid gland, however, is examined separately.

General observations
Some features of thyroid disease may be immediately detectable. These include the eye signs of Graves' disease, the goitre itself, and hoarseness. This should not dissuade the examiner from carrying out a full and systematic assessment. The examination is best approached in two stages as follows:

The gland and its surroundings
The neck should be inspected from the front. If a swelling is visible and lies in the region of the thyroid gland, ask the patient to swallow. (It is traditional to offer a glass of water, but not always essential.) A lump in the thyroid will move up on swallowing. Metastases to cervical lymph nodes may result in visible lumps lateral to the thyroid gland itself.

The gland is best palpated with the patient sitting and the examiner standing behind (226). The left hand can be used to retract the left sternomastoid muscle laterally, enabling the right hand to explore the left lobe. The roles of the two hands are reversed to examine the right lobe. The aim is to define the overall size and consistency of the swelling, and of the normal part of the gland if any. Can you 'get below' the gland, or does it appear to extend retrosternally (227)?

Diffuse nodular swelling suggests a multinodular goitre. A localized swelling may well be a prominent nodule in a multinodular goitre, but also raises the possibility of a cyst, adenoma, or malignant tumour. The fact that the swelling arises in the gland may be confirmed by asking the patient to swallow once again.

It is usual to palpate the regional lymph nodes and the trachea at this stage. The deep cervical lymph nodes lie adjacent to the carotid sheath, behind the anterior border of the sternomastoid muscle.

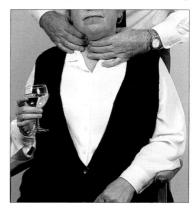

226 Palpation of thyroid.

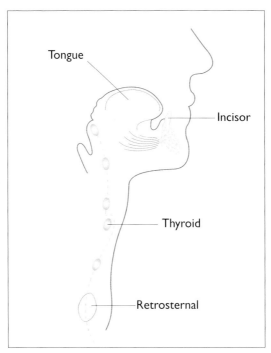

227 Descent of thyroid.

Supraclavicular lymph nodes and those in the posterior triangle of the neck (behind the sternomastoid muscle) should also be palpated. It is easiest to palpate the trachea when standing in front of the patient (see Chapter 3). Deviation to one side or other suggests a large retrosternal extension of the goitre. Percussion over the sternum may be performed, but it is not a reliable way of detecting retrosternal extension. Auscultation of the gland may reveal a bruit in patients with Graves' disease, but beware of transmitted cardiac murmurs or carotid bruits.

Other endocrine examinations
The common symptoms and signs associated with alterations in hormonal function are shown on the following pages. These are intended as a guide and not as a comprehensive account of endocrinology.

Hormonal dysfunction – symptoms and signs

Hormonal abnormality	Symptoms	Specific physical signs
Gonadotrophin deficiency		
Male	Fatigue, muscle weakness, loss of libido/sex drive; failure to sustain an erection	Delayed puberty. In adult: loss of facial, body, and pubertal hair; small and soft testes
Female	Irregular menses – amenorrhoea	Delayed menarche. In adult: often no specific signs
Growth hormone deficiency		
Children	Delayed growth	Short stature with obesity
Adults	Symptoms of associated pituitary hormone deficiencies	Obesity
Growth hormone excess		
Pre-fusion of the epiphysis: gigantism	Tallness with rapid increase in height	Excessive height
Post-fusion: acromegaly	Change in appearance, increase in size of hands and feet, headaches, weight gain. Excessive perspiration, joint pains	Characteristic acromegalic facies, large tongue, prominent supraorbital ridge, board nose, prognathism of lower jaw, thick greasy skin, spade-like hands, carpal tunnel syndrome
Thyroid hormone		
Thyroid deficiency (hypothyroidism)	Tiredness, malaise, weight gain, cold intolerance, change in appearance, dry skin, constipation	Mental slowness, dry thin hair, hypothermia, puffy eyes, loss of outer third of eyebrows, deep voice, obesity, slow relaxing reflexes; in primary thyroid failure – goitre

Hormonal abnormality	Symptoms	Specific physical signs
Thyroid excess (hyperthyroidism)	Weight loss, increased appetite, irritability, restlessness, tremor, palpitations, heat intolerance, diarrhoea, eye complaints, oligomenorrhoea	Exophthalmos, ophthalmoplegia, goitre with overlying bruit, weight loss, myopathy, brisk tendon reflexes, and wide tachycardia pulse pressure
Glucocorticoid axis		
Hyperadrenalism: Cushing's syndrome	Weight gain (upper body), change in appearance, thin skin with easy bruising, poor libido/menstrual abnormalities, hirsutism, acne, muscle weakness	Thin skin and bruising, moon face, plethora, buffalo hump, centripetal obesity, hypertension, proximal myopathy
Hypoadrenalism: Addison's disease	Weight loss, anorexia, impotence/amenorrhoea, nausea and vomiting, dizziness on standing, abdominal pain	Buccal and skin pigmentation, general wasting and loss of weight, postural hypotension, vitiligo may be associated
Arginine-vasopressin		
AVP/ADH excess: syndrome of inappropriate ADH (SIADH)	Symptoms resulting from hyponatraemia: headache, anorexia, irritability, lethargy. Extreme levels of hyponatraemia (Na <110 mmol/l) may be associated with drowsiness and fits	There may be no specific signs but may be accompanied by mental confusion and altered level of consciousness

… Continued overleaf

Hormonal abnormality	Symptoms	Specific physical signs
AVP/ADH deficiency	Excessive thirst and polyuria with passage of large volumes of urine; patients often relate how they require a jug of water by the bedside at night. Rarely presents with severe hypernatraemia and associated neurological confusion, fits and coma	No specific features but may be accompanied by signs of pituitary failure. Occasionally presents with dehydration with evidence of hypovolaemia (low blood pressure with postural fall)

Parathyroid hormone

Hyperparathyroidism	Personality change (often associated with depression), abdominal pain – constipation and/or dyspepsia, polyuria and polydipsia	Severe and prolonged hypercalcaemia, may be accompanied by corneal calcification, associated hypertension, haematuria if associated with renal calculi
Hypoparathyroidism	Paraesthesia, cramps, alterations in personality (occasionally psychosis), epilepsy	Carpopedal spasm (positive Trousseau's sign), positive Chvostek's sign (twitching of facial muscle on tapping), cataract formation

Insulin

Insulin deficiency: diabetes mellitus	May present in any age group. Symptoms resulting from hyperglycaemia include thirst, polyuria, weight loss and intense fatigue, recurrent skin infections. Patients may also have related complaints: impotence, paraesthesia/ hypoasthesia of hands/feet, visual disturbances, and foot ulcers	Look for signs of complications: examine the fundi to look for retinal changes, examine the feet to detect any loss of sensation (light touch, pinprick, and vibrations sense). Examine pulses in lower limbs and test urine for protein and glucose

Hormonal abnormality	Symptoms	Specific physical signs
Insulin excess: hypoglycaemia	Patient may present in a coma. Symptoms suggestive of hypoglycaemia include hunger, cold perspiration, tremor, pallor, and agitation. Generalized convulsion may accompany profound hypoglycaemia	Severe hypoglycaemia may present with focal neurological signs (reversible if glucose quickly restored to normal). Usually, the patient is cold and clammy with a 'bounding' pulse and a moderately elevated blood pressure

Illustrated physical signs

The following photographs illustrate some common endocrine physical signs: a large, multinodular goitre (228); thyrotoxicosis (229); Addison's disease (230); acromegaly (231); and Cushing's syndrome (232).

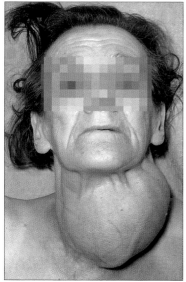

228 A large multinodular goitre.

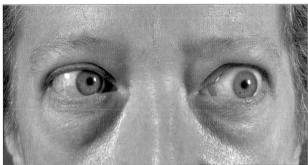

229 Thyrotoxicosis causing lid retraction and dysconjugate gaze from thyroid eye disease.

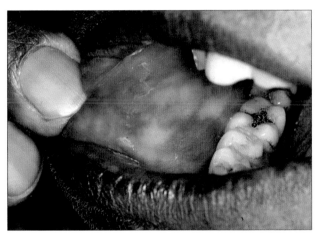

230 Buccal pigmentation in Addison's disease.

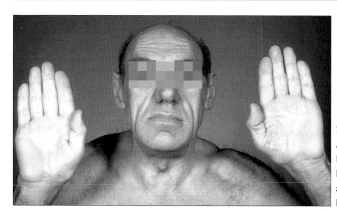

231
Acromegaly.
Note the
lantern jaw
and wide
hands.

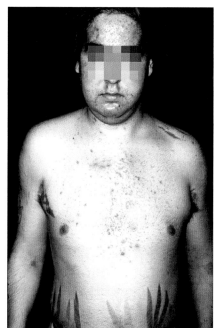

232 Cushing's syndrome
with central obesity, acne,
and striae.

Figures **233** and **234** highlight common findings in hyper- and hypothyroidism, respectively.

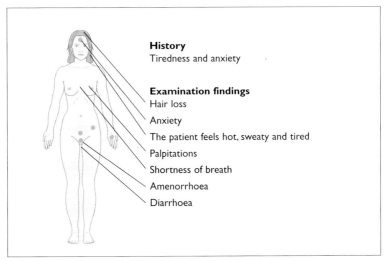

History
Tiredness and anxiety

Examination findings
Hair loss

Anxiety

The patient feels hot, sweaty and tired

Palpitations

Shortness of breath

Amenorrhoea

Diarrhoea

233 Hyperthyroidism.

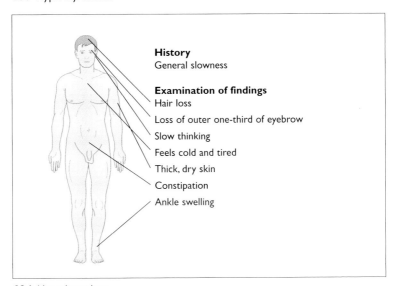

History
General slowness

Examination of findings
Hair loss

Loss of outer one-third of eyebrow

Slow thinking

Feels cold and tired

Thick, dry skin

Constipation

Ankle swelling

234 Hypothyroidism.

10 The skin

The skin is an important physiological structure. It also has a significant effect on a patient's psychological well-being, as dermatological diseases often cause blemishes and abnormalities which, although minor, may be a very large problem to the patient.

Applied anatomy of the skin

The skin consists of two layers:

- An outer epidermis: this is composed of keratinized stratified squamous epithelium. Hair follicles, sweat glands, sebaceous glands, and nails are modifications of the epidermis.
- An inner dermis: this is vascular connective tissue, containing tubular sweat ducts opening on to the skin's surface, and sebaceous glands opening on the hair follicles. The roots of hair and sweat glands are present in the subcutaneous tissue.

The anatomy of skin is illustrated in **235**.

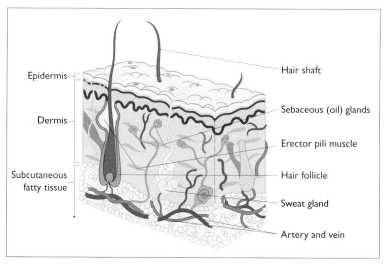

Epidermis

Dermis

Subcutaneous fatty tissue

Hair shaft

Sebaceous (oil) glands

Erector pili muscle

Hair follicle

Sweat gland

Artery and vein

235 Anatomy of skin.

Assessment and diagnosis

The structure of the dermatological history is the same as for any other system, but dermatological conditions frequently have a pattern recognition element, and can be made as spot diagnoses.

Taking the history

The presenting complaint

The patient may complain of a 'rash', 'spots', 'itching', an 'ulcer', or a 'growth'. It is important to ask them to describe exactly what they are worried about, and also to describe the distribution of the abnormality. Also ask about provoking and alleviating factors such as hot, cold, warm, or dry conditions. Ask:

● 'Is the condition spreading or does it look as though it is gradually improving?'

Although often quite difficult, it is important to find out how long a rash or skin problem has been present. This is particularly true of skin tumours. It is also important to find out what has happened to a lesion since it started. Has it spread from the centre or from the edge or has it come in crops and occasionally disappeared?

Past medical history

It is worthwhile asking whether the patient has had previous skin problems, as these may have been present since birth.

Social history

An occupational history is very important in skin disease, as several chemicals used in industry can irritate the skin or give rise to allergy. Remember that skin allergies can also be provoked by hobbies, rashes can be provoked by plant antigens, and it is also important to ask about sunlight. Short-term exposure to the sun can precipitate photosensitive rashes, sometimes associated with drug reactions. In addition, repeated exposure over several years predisposes to rodent ulcers, squamous cell carcinoma, and malignant melanoma.

Family history

It is important to establish whether there is a family history of atopy in patients with eczema, and of psoriasis in patients who you suspect have a psoriatic rash. Other less common skin complaints also have a familial link, e.g. porphyria cutanea tarda.

Drug history

It is essential to establish which drugs patients are taking, and for how long. Drugs are an important cause of a large number of eruptions. Remember that some drugs may have been taken for some months before a rash appears, e.g. gold or penicillamine in rheumatoid arthritis.

Examination of the patient
Examination of the skin is largely based on inspection. The lesions should be identified and described. Any secondary changes such as excoriation should be established and documented. The shape, size, colour, and consistency of any lesions should also be clearly documented, and their distribution over the skin noted. In addition, it is important to carry out a general examination, as skin conditions are often a component of a multisystem disorder.

Key features of skin disease
It is particularly important not to miss the changes in a mole that may suggest malignant transformation. These are: a change in shape; variability in colour; size >1 cm; bleeding; and itching.

Lesions to look for especially include benign pigmented naevus (236), atypical mole (237), malignant melanoma (238), and basal cell carcinoma (239).

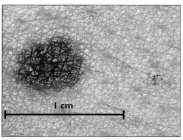

236 Pigmented naevus.

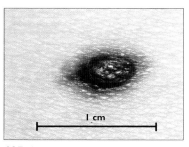

237 Atypical mole.

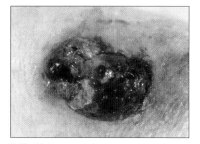

238 Malignant melanoma.

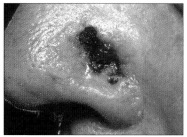

239 Basal cell carcinoma.

Illustrated physical signs

This section includes clinical photographs of common dermatological conditions: vitiligo (240); atopic eczema (241); psoriasis of the elbow (242); psoriasis of the sole of the foot (243); acne (244); xanthelasma (245); butterfly rash of SLE (246); and vasculitic rash (247).

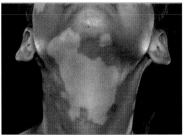

240 Vitiligo.

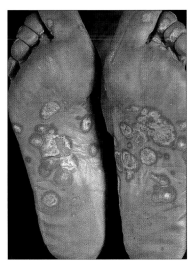

241 Atopic eczema.

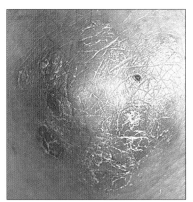

242 Psoriasis of the elbow.

243 Psoriasis of the soles of the feet.

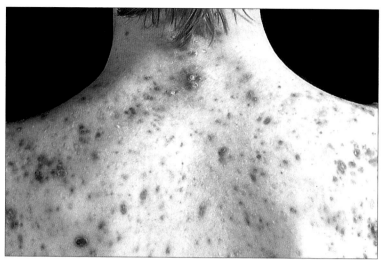

244 Acne.

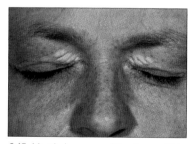

245 Xanthelasma, resulting from a high level of cholesterol in the blood.

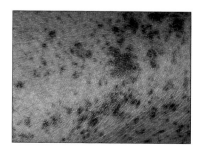

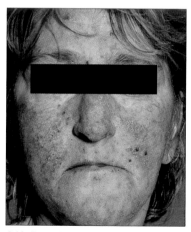

246 Butterfly rash in systemic lupus erythematosus.

247 Vasculitic rash.

Common definitions in skin conditions

Dermatology, as with any other speciality, has its own group of descriptive terms. Fortunately these are few and easy to remember:

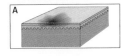

A Macule – a flat spot of a different colour from the surrounding skin, e.g. freckles.

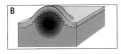

B Papule – a raised spot on the surface of the skin. **Nodule** – usually indicates a lump deeply set in the skin.

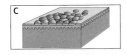

C Scale – a flake of flat horny cells loosened from the horny layer.

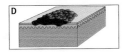

D Crust – a deeply situated, fluid-filled cavity.

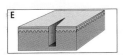

E Fissure – a crack or split.

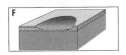

F Erosion – an area of partial loss of skin or mucous membrane.

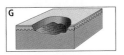

G Ulcer – an area of total loss of epithelium of skin or mucous membrane.

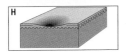

H Atrophy – loss of thickness.

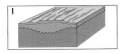

I Lichenification – thickening.

Common definitions in skin conditions

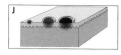

J Vesicle – a small blister, e.g. herpes simplex.
Blister (bulla) – a skin bleb with clear fluid. It may be subepidermal, e.g. pemphigoid and dermatitis herpetiformis, or intra-epidermal, e.g. pemphigus, eczema.

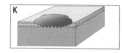

K Excoriation – a scratch mark that has scored the epidermis.

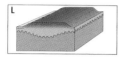

L Plaque – a raised uniform thickening of a portion of the skin with a well-defined edge and a flat or rough surface, e.g. psoriasis.

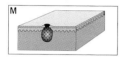

M Comedone – an accumulation of keratin and sebum lodged in the dilated pilosebaceous orifice.

N Erythema – redness.

The following illustrations highlight the distribution of lesions in common skin conditions: psoriasis (248), acne (249), and seborrhoeic dermatitis (250).

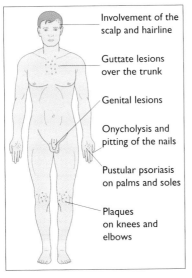

Involvement of the scalp and hairline

Guttate lesions over the trunk

Genital lesions

Onycholysis and pitting of the nails

Pustular psoriasis on palms and soles

Plaques on knees and elbows

248 Psoriasis.

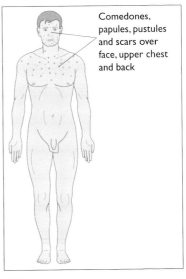

Comedones, papules, pustules and scars over face, upper chest and back

249 Acne.

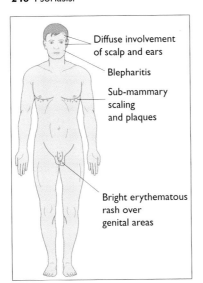

Diffuse involvement of scalp and ears

Blepharitis

Sub-mammary scaling and plaques

Bright erythematous rash over genital areas

250 Seborrhoeic dermatitis.

11 Psychiatric assessment of the patient

All doctors should be able to undertake a psychiatric assessment, as patients with psychiatric symptoms are commonly encountered in all branches of medicine. Psychiatry is concerned with the study and management of patients with disorders of mental functions. Such conditions are believed to arise as a result of a combination of physical (genetic, neurochemical), psychological, and social factors. Rather than being based on an established aetiology, psychiatric diagnosis depends on recognition of groups of symptoms (syndromes), which occur consistently and, to a certain extent, predict response to specific treatments. Diagnosis not only helps in planning treatment but also facilitates communication and research. This chapter will focus on the clinical skills involved in the assessment of patients with psychiatric disorders. Accurate diagnosis depends on knowledge of the symptoms associated with the various psychiatric disorders, interview skills, and the ability to collect information in a clear and systematic manner.

Symptoms and classification of mental illness

Psychiatric symptoms are often associated with subjective distress or impairment of function which leads the individual to seek help. They may also be identified by a change in behaviour which puts the person at risk, or becomes a problem to others. Some symptoms in psychiatry vary in degree from feelings associated with normal human experience, but at their worst can be extremely disabling. They are sometimes referred to as neurotic symptoms and include, for example, anxious and depressed mood. The term 'psychotic' may be applied to symptoms which differ in quality from normal experience. Insight is often impaired, and they can have a major impact on the individual's functioning. Examples include delusions and hallucinations (see page 278, 'Mental state examination'). These symptoms are associated with conditions such as delirium and schizophrenia, which may be referred to as psychoses. This distinction is reflected in the classification of psychiatric disorders into categories based on what are believed to be the central symptoms. A hierarchy is implied whereby certain diagnoses take precedence if symptoms are evident to suggest more than one. The order of precedence is as listed (**Table 32**). If, for example, there are symptoms to suggest schizophrenia in the presence of significant anxiety symptoms, then the primary diagnosis is schizophrenia.

There is no ideal system of classification, in the absence of biological markers of disease (**Table 32**). Although some symptoms can suggest certain conditions, others are less specific and can occur across a range of disorders. Furthermore, there is variation within each diagnostic category. Mood disorders may range from mild to severe forms, with different symptoms. Schizophrenia can be considered to be a heterogeneous spectrum of disorders of variable presentation and outcome.

Table 32. Examples of different types of psychiatric disorder

Main adult psychiatric diagnoses

- Organic mental disorders
    - Acute (delirium)
    - Chronic (dementia)
- Psychoactive substance use disorders
- Schizophrenic and related disorders
- Affective (mood) disorders
    - Depressive disorders
    - Mania
- Neurotic disorders
    - Anxiety disorders
    - Phobic disorders
    - Reactions to stress
    - Obsessional compulsive disorder
    - Dissociative disorders
    - Somatoform disorders (e.g. pain syndromes, unexplained physical symptoms)
    - Eating disorders
    - Sexual disorders
- Personality disorders
- Learning disabilities

The presenting complaint

It is useful to start by explaining the purpose of the interview, how it will proceed, and by addressing any initial questions that the patient may have. Begin with open general questions to identify the most significant concerns:

● 'Could you tell me about some of the problems that led to your coming to see me?'

● 'How have you been feeling?'

Try to allow the patient to talk freely and without interruption for a few minutes. If the patient appears unaware of any specific problems or finds talking difficult, refer to other available information.

'I have a letter from your GP which says you've been having some difficulties concerning ... could you tell me some more about this?'

Identify each complaint, and record it in the patient's own words. For each, attempt to clarify:

● Time of onset. Be as specific as possible. 'When did you first become aware of this problem?' or 'When were you last reasonably well?'

Antecedents or precipitants. 'Did anything happen or change just before this problem began?' Some examples may be given to the patient. 'Were you feeling physically unwell ... were you under a lot of stress ... were there any difficulties at home or work?' Establish whether any such difficulties preceded, or may have resulted from, psychological symptoms.

● Mode of onset and time course. Determine whether the symptoms developed suddenly or gradually and have remained persistent. Enquire about any periods of respite, reduction, or intensification, and if anything is associated with relief or exacerbation.

● Time relations between different symptoms. Enquire about the sequence of events from the time the patient reported last being well, in order to identify which symptoms came first, and which may have arisen subsequently. If there are a number of complaints, their time of onset in relation to each other can be important for diagnosis, e.g. anxiety symptoms or persecutory feelings following other symptoms of depression.

● Associated symptoms. The patient's initial complaints may indicate other areas of enquiry. In most cases, it is appropriate to ask direct brief screening questions for symptoms of anxiety, depression, suicidal ideas, hostile feelings toward others, or psychotic phenomena (see page 276, 'Mental state examination'), but this will depend on the individual case.

● Effects on usual level of functioning. Symptoms of psychiatric disorders often impair an individual's functioning, which in turn reflects the severity of the condition. Enquiring about sleep pattern, appetite, weight change, sexual function, and self care often reveals abnormalities which can support certain diagnoses. Waking earlier than usual, reduced appetite and weight, decreased libido, and diurnal variation in mood (lower in the morning) suggests depression of at least moderate severity. These symptoms are often called biological. In mania, in which the mood is elevated, sleeping time is reduced without tiredness and libido may increase.

Assessment and diagnosis of psychiatric disorder

Taking the history
The psychiatric interview
A good interview technique takes time to develop, but is central to good psychiatric practice. The clinical interview is used for the following purposes:
- Establishing trust.
- Gathering information.
- Making a diagnosis.
- Therapeutic, as many patients find it helpful to talk their problems through.

Setting Interviews should be carried out in circumstances that allow privacy. Preferably, this will be in a room free from interruptions or distractions. Chairs should be arranged at an angle, and interviewing across a desk avoided.

Personal safety Personal safety should always be considered, although overall it is unusual for patients with mental illness to be violent. If you have any concerns, other members of staff should be within earshot, or should accompany you. Ideally, there should be a panic button to hand, and you should sit between the patient and the exit to the room. If it is felt that a patient will be violent, it is advisable politely to terminate the interview, leave, and summon help.

Assessment
The process of assessment begins from the moment the patient is first encountered, at which stage important observations can be made before any verbal exchanges. Information collected should be clear, and recorded systematically.

Informants Although the patient is the main source of information, it is always helpful to have information from other individuals whose knowledge would add to an understanding of the patient's difficulties. Such corroborating informants would include other professionals, family, and friends. This should be sought preferably with the patient's consent, and is particularly important if the patient denies any problem, or if the assessment has been arranged in response to concerns expressed by others. Such information should be identified clearly and recorded separately. The information that follows should be sought and recorded.

Table 33. Important areas of inquiry
• Main concerns
• Mood symptoms
• Delusions
• Hallucinations

Family history

The purpose of this section of the history is to identify significant predisposing factors, and to assess current support or family stresses. There is evidence for a significant genetic contribution to some of the major mental illnesses, and intra-familial childhood relationships can predispose to later problems. Ask about:

• Father and mother: for each, ask about their age, occupation, physical and psychiatric health (including alcohol or other substance misuse), temperament, nature of the relationship with the patient in the past and presently, and the quality of the parents' own inter-relationship. Try to assess the validity of the answers given by reflecting the patient's feelings and asking open, exploratory questions.

• Siblings: ask about ages, order of birth, occupations, marital status, nature of relationship in the past and present, and their physical and psychiatric health.

• Separations or disruptions, e.g. marital break-up, relationship with step-parent.

• Adverse recollections and attitude to childhood.

• Atmosphere in the family home.

• Important adult figures, e.g. a teacher, doctor.

Source and reason for referral This provides clues about the nature of the difficulties – which may not be initially apparent from the patient's account.

You should also ask about the effects on work, family commitments (e.g. child-care), relationships, and social activities. It is helpful to ask the patient to describe the activities of a typical day at present, and then describe a typical day before to the onset of their difficulties.

Previous help Ask about any other treatment during the course of their current problems and their response. Record current and recently taken medication.

Past psychiatric history

Establish whether the patient has ever had psychiatric problems before and ask about previous diagnoses or treatments with their nature, response, and duration. Determine the similarity to current symptoms and the extent of recovery from previous episodes. Always ask about episodes of self-harm.

Previous history should also include:

- Episodes for which no assistance was sought.
- GP consultations.
- Psychiatric assessments and admissions. Try to obtain previous records; ask about regular medication, e.g. depot antipsychotic preparations.

Past medical history

Medical conditions and their treatments can give rise to psychiatric disorders, and possible drug interactions must be considered when prescribing psychotropic medication. Enquiries should be made concerning:

- Acute and chronic medical illness, e.g. epilepsy, diabetes, carcinoma.
- Medication both prescribed (e.g. steroids) and self-administered (e.g. diet pills).
- Major surgery, head injuries.

Background history

It helps to explain to patients that background information can contribute to an understanding of their current difficulties, before beginning a detailed enquiry. Although the majority of patients are able to talk about personal details of their lives without too much difficulty, some may be uncomfortable during the first interview. The areas covered are slightly different from the usual areas in a medical or surgical history, and include both family and personal sexual histories, a forensic history, details of any substance misuse, and personality.

Sexual abuse Childhood sexual abuse can be difficult to discuss, and may require time. This can be approached using a question such as, 'When you were growing up did anyone ever hurt or abuse you ... was this ever physical or sexual?'

Women may suffer significant psychiatric symptoms premenstrually or around the time of the menopause, as well as postnatally or following a termination. It is important to ask about possible pregnancy before prescribing. Antipsychotic medication can cause amenorrhoea and galactorrhoea – a fact which is less distressing if it is explained. Areas covered may include regularity, dysmenorrhoea, menorrhagia, last period, premenstrual syndrome (physical

Personal history

A chronological account of the important events from birth to the present should obtained, covering:

● Childhood: enquiries may reveal causes and evidence of learning disabilities or longstanding behaviour problems.

● Birth and neonatal history: health, e.g. injuries/infections/convulsions. Developmental milestones (walking and talking).

● Education: this gives an indication of intelligence and development both social and emotional against which you can compare current functioning. In particular, relevant enquiries may cover the patient's schooling – 'Were there disruptions … was there any special education … were there conduct or emotional problems (e.g. school refusal)?' Also, ask about relationships with peers and teachers, bullying, truancy, participation in social activities, academic performance-specific difficulties (e.g. reading), and general attitude to school. Determine the age at which the patient left school, their qualifications, and further education.

● Occupation: the patient's work record can add to an understanding of their personality and capabilities, as well as to the onset and severity of mental health problems. Current work or unemployment may be a significant stress. Discrepancies between education and employment record, or a decline in responsibilities, may reflect functional impairment suggesting repeated or chronic mental illness. Important information includes the duration of employment and reasons for termination, attitude to work, satisfaction, performance, and relationships with employers and colleagues.

and psychological symptoms and treatment), pregnancies (including miscarriages, terminations, and stillbirths), and subsequent psychiatric problems, menopausal symptoms, and treatment.

Sexual history

Enquiries about sexual behaviour should be approached with discretion. A more detailed account is required if there is a sexual problem. Establishing how comfortable the patient is with the questions and giving permission to decline to respond can put the patient more at ease.

'Do you mind if I ask about your sexual life/the physical side of your relationship?'

If it is explained that a number of psychiatric disorders (e.g. anxiety, depression) and their treatments are associated with alterations in libido and sexual functions, most patients will appreciate the opportunity for discussion. Sexual problems can add considerably to the distress of psychiatric disorders, and can be an unexpressed reason for non-compliance with psychotropic medication.

'It's not uncommon for the problems you describe to affect your sexual life. Have you noticed any changes?'

'Have there been any difficulties on the physical side of the relationship?'

Areas covered may include:

- Sexual development and current practice.
- Satisfaction.
- Dysfunction.
- Contraceptive measures, and safe sexual practice.
- Sexually transmissible diseases.

Relationships, marriage, and children The course, duration, and quality of relationships can reflect personality, and suggest areas of stress. Mental health problems may be caused by or impair relationships. It is important to ask about children and their problems. Enquiries include:

- Current status: e.g. married/cohabiting, duration, partner's personality and occupation, quality and satisfaction, attitude toward partner, e.g. separations, ability to confide or communicate, give and receive support.
- Previous relationships: age of first significant relationship, subsequent relationships (details as above, focusing on the most important), longest within and outside relationship, any repeated patterns within relationships, reasons for ending, e.g. divorce, death of spouse, dates and patient's response.
- Children: names, health, learning or behavioural problems, psychiatric help, ability to provide care, attitudes to children, quality of relationship, social services involvement, and family composition.

Current life circumstances Ask which life circumstances, if any, cause undue stress. If none is identified, then enquiries about money, housing, neighbours, and support of family, friends, or professional agencies may identify significant stresses, or areas of need.

Forensic history

This may be a sensitive area, and the purpose of questions should be explained clearly. If a report is to be prepared, the patient often needs to give consent. Your questions may identify longstanding maladaptive behaviour or legal transgressions driven by symptoms of psychiatric illness.

- 'Have you had any difficulties which led to legal problems or contact with the police?'
- 'Have you ever been accused of any offence?'

Particularly note any violent or sexual offences, or other dangerous behaviour (e.g. arson).

This will have implications for management and for the safety of others, including those involved in the patient's care. Even if there has been no legal involvement, you should ask about previous aggressive behaviour in order to gain an impression of the level of dangerousness of which the patient has been capable. Recognition of any changes in the pattern of offences or the onset of offending behaviour at a particular time may suggest a psychiatric illness.

You should ask about arrests, convictions and detentions, longest period of imprisonment, mental health detentions via the courts or prison, attitude to offending behaviour, probation and probation officer, outstanding charges.

Substance misuse Substances differ in their abilities to cause dependence and withdrawal symptoms, and in their tendency to precipitate psychiatric symptoms. Patients may present with symptoms reflecting drug intoxication, withdrawal, or with psychiatric disorders triggered by the abuse of drugs. The acute effects of drugs may include psychotic symptoms (seen most often with amphetamine, cocaine, and LSD). Alcohol abuse is associated with delirium tremens, chronic organic brain disorders, and a chronic paranoid psychosis. If drug abuse is suspected, urine samples should be screened.

Enquiries should include :

- The substance used, the duration of first use, route of administration, and use of safe injecting practice.
- The amount used. This is sometimes difficult to clarify. Ask how much was used in the previous day, and work backwards to build up a picture of use during the previous week initially. Ask how much is spent and how the habit is funded.
- Evidence of dependence, the longest period of abstinence, withdrawal (e.g. alcohol – morning nausea or shaking, delirium tremens, fits).
- Adverse effects – psychological, physical, social (e.g. criminality, family, or work problems).
- Treatments – e.g. outpatient/inpatient detoxification, rehabilitation, Alcoholics Anonymous.

Personality This describes an individual's habitual pattern of behaviour. It is important not to stereotype your patient, or be judgemental about a patient's personality. A personality disorder occurs when a person's consistent behaviour causes repeated suffering to him/herself or to other people. This disorder is different from a mental illness by there being no clear onset, and by the longstanding nature of the problems which usually start in childhood or adolescence. Personality may influence the expression of mental illness. Furthermore, stresses which can precipitate illness can also exacerbate the maladaptive behaviour which characterizes personality disorders.

Table 34. Assessment of deliberate self-harm

Common presentation. The aim is to identify mental illness and patients at risk of completing suicide. Factors associated with increased risk include:

The patient
- Socially isolated
- Male
- Older age (young males also higher risk)
- Unemployed

The attempt
- Planning, e.g. taking care of affairs, leaving note, steps to avoid detection
- Method. e.g. violent, severe (if overdose), or believed to be lethal

The history
- Recent life event, e.g. bereavement, retirement, divorce
- Psychiatric diagnosis
- Previous attempt(s)
- Chronic painful illness
- Family history of mental illness/suicide
- Alcohol or drug misuse

Mental state
- Depressed mood
- Suicidal thoughts
- Hopelessness
- Delusions/hallucinations

In assessing personality sources of information include:

- The patient's account – this may be coloured by the current illness, e.g. depressed patients may have difficulty saying anything positive about themselves. It may also be inaccurate, e.g. antisocial behaviour may be understated, or a report of being 'happy-go-lucky' given when this trait is not corroborated.
- Moods, stability/variability ('cyclothymia').
- Impulse control, e.g. self-harm, verbal or physical aggression (see **Table 34**).
- Leisure, solitary or collective, hobbies, interests.

- Stress coping, how previous difficulties were dealt with.
- Information from other parts of the history may provide a better indication of any problems, e.g. adversity, suffering, behavioural, or emotional problems in early life, relationship or work difficulties, antisocial behaviour (e.g. criminality or substance misuse).
- Objective opinions of other informants who know the patient well are often the most reliable sources of information. It is important to obtain the patient's consent first, if possible.

The following areas of enquiry may be relevant :

- Attitude to others and to self, e.g. friends, colleagues, ability to trust and confide, self-esteem, confidence, self-consciousness, satisfaction with achievements.
- Standards, e.g. religious beliefs, obsessionality, perfectionism.

Questions may include: 'How would you describe yourself?... What do you feel are your strengths and weaknesses?'

A number of traits associated with defined personality disorders have been described. Examples include anankastic (obsessional), passive-dependent, passive-aggressive, anti-social, and paranoid. It is best to describe patients using dimensional measures (e.g. 'moderately passive aggressive') rather than categorical descriptions, as there is considerable overlap between personality traits, and the severity of a disorder will determine its presentation. A checklist for psychiatric history taking is shown in Table 35.

Table 35. Checklist for history taking

- Demographic information
- Presenting complaints
- Past psychiatric history
- Past medical history
- Family history
- Personal background
  - Childhood
  - Education
  - Occupation
  - Sexual and relationships
  - Current social circumstances
- Forensic history
- Substance misuse
- Personality

Examination of the patient
Mental state examination

The mental state examination (MSE) is an assessment of the patient's behaviour and state of mind at the time of the interview (Table 36). It is analogous to the physical examination in general medicine. While the history can be expanded subsequent to the initial assessment, the MSE is a once-only 'snapshot' taken at a particular time. Repeated examinations may be needed as part of the diagnostic process, so that a patient can explain and better communicate their internal world, as well as respond to changing thoughts and feelings. The MSE may be the only source of information on which to base the initial diagnosis and management, for example in the case of uncooperative or uncom-municative patients.

A good MSE depends on good use of communication skills and knowledge of how key symptoms are defined (descriptive psychopathology), asking appropriate questions, and systematic collection of information under the headings outlined. Clear descriptions and quoted speech are preferable to subjective terms such as 'normal' or 'reasonable', which convey little information. Negative findings may be recorded if this contributes to the diagnosis or management, e.g. no depressive affect or no suicidal ideas. Information from corroborative sources, e.g. nursing observations, may be included.

Table 36. Mental state examination
● Appearance and behaviour
● Speech
● Mood
● Thought content
● Perception
● Cognitive function
● Insight

Appearance and behaviour

This section of the examination can provide important clues to diagnosis, as a great deal of subjective mental experience can be reflected in the patient's appearance and behaviour. However, be careful not to be judgemental in your assessment.

Aspects to consider include general physical appearance, state of dress, facial appearance, posture and movement (gait), and socially interactive behaviour. The attitude to the interviewer, rapport, and level of cooperation will be variable. Some of the observable features which may reflect psychiatric problems include:

- **Anxiety:** tension, apprehension, sensitivity to noise or light, vigilance, irritability, restlessness, tendency to fidget. Face – flushed or pale, sweating, lined due to tension in the facial muscles. Eyes – widened, pupils dilated. Posture – stiff, tense, elevated shoulders.
- **Depression:** Poor self-care, signs of weight loss, difficult rapport. Face – sad, unanimated, reduced blinking, tears. Eyes – contact reduced, eyes down-cast. Reduced or increased movement (retardation or agitation).
- **Mania:** over-activity, disinhibition, distractability, noisiness, irritability, arousal, over-friendliness or familiarity, hostility, or truculence. Clothes – bright, inappropriate, or neglected. Face – cheerful or irritated look. Eye contact: intense.

- **Hallucinating:** strange, seemingly purposeless behaviour, sudden changes in movements, cooperation and attention reduced, distracted, socially withdrawn. Face – preoccupied or perplexed, sudden intense change in gaze in response to extraneous stimuli, unusual movements of the facial muscles, sub-vocal movements of the mouth or tongue, talking to self, incongruous smiling or fear.
- **Delusions:** bizarre behaviour, arousal, hostility due to suspiciousness, verbal or physical aggression. Dress – bizarre or inappropriate. Face – fearful and wary. Eyes scanning the environment.
- **Delirium:** impaired attention, reduced cooperation, over-activity alternating with inactivity, repetitive purposeless movements (plucking at the bed-clothes). Signs of anxiety, hallucinations, and abnormal ideas.
- **Schizophrenia:** strange, inappropriate, or socially awkward behaviour, self-neglect. Behaviour suggesting delusions or hallucinations. Blunted or absent affect. Uncommon specific motor abnormalities may be evident which include stereotypies (repeated regular movements without obvious purpose, e.g. rocking to-and-fro), mannerisms (regular movements with some functional significance, e.g. saluting), posturing (adopting bodily positions for long periods of time), negativism (a tendency to perform the opposite action to that which is asked while resisting efforts to encourage compliance), waxy flexibility (limbs may be placed into positions in which they remain for long periods, associated with a feeling of plastic resistance), echopraxia (automatic imitation of interviewer's movements), ambitendence (seemingly purposeless alternation between opposite movements). There may be signs of side-effects of medication, e.g. akathisia, pseudo-Parkinson's, or tardive dyskinesia (involuntary orofacial or bodily movements).

Speech

This section deals with how the patient speaks, which is assessed with reference to tone, volume, spontaneity, rate, quantity (amount), and form (reflecting the form of thought).

- In **depression**, speech may be monotonous and softly delivered, hesitant or only in response to questions (reduced spontaneity). The rate may be reduced (retardation of speech) which, together with slow movement, are described as psychomotor retardation. Speech may be reduced in amount and monosyllabic (poverty of speech).

- In **mania**, speech may be loud, rapid, and difficult to interrupt (pressure of speech). Speech may be disordered in the form of flight of ideas, which is characterized by frequent shifts of topic connected by sounds, puns, rhymes, or word associations, which can be difficult to follow. Other abnormalities of the form of speech include circumstantial (inability to stick to the point), neologisms (new words created by patient), and perseveration (repetition of the previous verbal response).
- **Thought blocking** is an abrupt cessation in the flow of speech which can be experienced when anxious, but may be a manifestation of delusional experience (i.e. thought withdrawal – see below). If this occurs, ask why – 'Could you tell me what happened when you suddenly stopped talking?'
- **Disordered thinking** occurs with schizophrenia. The speech becomes difficult to understand or unintelligible, and the logical sequence of thoughts is difficult to follow. This is also referred to as 'loosening of associations' or 'knight's move thinking'. In its most severe form, speech becomes an incoherent mixture of words and phrases ('word salad').

Mood/affect

Change in mood defines a mood disorder, but may also occur in other psychiatric disorders. Objective evidence of mood disturbance can be taken from the patient's appearance, behaviour and speech, and is termed his/her 'affect'. A patient will describe his/her mood and will feel an emotion. Examine for:

- **Congruity:** does the affect match the patient's described mood? Incongruity suggests loss of control over emotional responses and can be seen in schizophrenia and personality disorders.
- **Reactivity:** this refers to how the mood changes during the interview as a response to the social interaction.

Specific mood disturbances

These include:

- Depressed, whereby the mood is reported as sad, low, despondent, anhedonic (lacking enjoyment), blue.
- Elevated, described as extraordinarily happy, high, elated, super-confident, full of energy – as seen in mania.
- Anxious, fearful, apprehensive, worrying repetitively.
- Irritable, with impatience, anger, hostility – as seen in both mania and depressive illness.
- Labile, where the mood rapidly changes from high to low and irritable, as seen in mania, mixed affective states (an uncommon mixture of depression and mania), and delirium.
- Blunted, where the mood is impassive or absent, as often seen in chronic schizophrenia.

Initial, open questions might be:

- 'How are you feeling?'
- 'How do you feel in your mood?'

Closed questions might include:

- 'Have you been feeling particularly low or sad ... happy or particularly cheerful?'

If the answer is yes, then ask for elaboration.

The extent of the mood disturbance and the thoughts that may develop from it must be explored by asking about the following. Abnormalities may be evident, even if mood disturbance is not conspicuous:

- **Biological features:** changes in sleep, appetite, weight, sexual function, bowel habit, and diurnal variation in mood – suggesting that depression may be identified from the history.
- **Motivation/interest:** if reduced, and the patient becomes less productive (depression). 'Have you found yourself motivated to do the things you usually do?' If increased – with over-activity, extravagant projects might be started, but not necessarily completed or well done (mania). 'Have you developed any new interests recently?'
- **Energy:** reduced (depression) or increased (mania).
- **Ability to experience pleasure:** an inability to experience pleasure (anhedonia) is an important symptom, which suggests significant depression of mood. Look for change in attitude to things that the patient previously enjoyed, taking examples from the history. 'Are you able to enjoy anything at the present time?'

- **Memory and concentration:** ask about subjective impairments which may be evident in depression.
- **Helplessness or hopelessness:** Loss of hope and pessimism indicates significantly depressed mood, and is a predictive factor for suicide. 'Do you see things improving?' … 'How do you see the future?'
- **Suicidal feelings:** if a depressed mood is suspected, then suicidal thoughts and any plans made must be explored in detail. Asking about the subject does not put new ideas into patient's heads. Those with suicidal thoughts (the majority of patients with depressive illness) will find that it helps to talk about these feelings. Identifying them shows an understanding and acknowledgement of the patient's distress. 'How bad does it get?' … 'Have you had any desperate thoughts?' … 'Have you thought it would be better not to go on?' … 'Have you had any suicidal thoughts or intent?'
- **Other mood-associated thoughts:** a negative attitude to him/herself, others and events, guilt, self-recrimination, worthlessness, and low self-esteem are all associated with depression. Over-confidence and excessive optimism, expansive thinking, and extravagant plans (see also delusions) are all associated with mania.

Thought content You should concentrate your enquiries on abnormalities suggesting diagnoses. These may include predominant concerns or morbid ideas. Record the patient's responses to questions such as: 'What would you say are your main worries?' Subsequent questions may be guided by the history. Specific enquiries may be necessary concerning:

- Anxiety, panic (sudden-onset intense fear and apprehension associated with physical symptoms of anxiety and ideas of 'losing control'), phobias (morbid irrational fears of situations or objects which are then avoided): 'Have you been feeling anxious, tense or frightened … how often? … under what circumstances?' 'Are you having these feelings now?'
- Attitude to health, bodily concern or body image disturbance: 'Have you any worries about your physical health?'
- Obsessions (recurrent persistent thoughts, impulses or images present despite efforts to resist them). These ruminations are recognized as the patient's own, and often concern dirt or contamination. They are usually associated with compulsive behaviour in order to minimize the ruminations (e.g. repeated hand washing.) 'Have you been finding decisions difficult?' 'Have you been spending a lot of time washing yourself or checking things?'

Delusions

These are beliefs for which there are no rational grounds, which are unshakeable despite counter-argument or proof to the contrary, and which are inconsistent with the cultural background.

Delusions are very helpful in making a diagnosis. Their presence defines the illness as a psychosis. Delusions may be detected when the patient is asked about main worries, but closed questions are often required. A positive response to such a question should always be clarified with open questions. The firmness with which the belief is held, and its plausibility, should be established. Ask the patient about the feelings which are associated with the abnormal beliefs expressed, and whether he/she has any particular actions in mind. Delusional thinking may motivate behaviour, and detailed enquiries should be made considering the health and safety of the patient and that of other people. Delusions may be classified according to the following:

Onset

Primary delusions are uncommon, but highly suggestive of schizophrenia. They arise from a delusional mood, and usually follow a delusional perception. A delusional mood is the feeling that something unusual and ill-defined is happening which concerns the patient. A delusional perception is a normal perception followed by a delusional interpretation.

- 'Do you have a feeling that something strange is going on around you?'
- 'Do you feel that some of the things you see around you have a particular meaning for you?'

Clarification is always required.

Secondary delusions arise out of previous morbid experience, e.g. delusions of guilt, following the onset of depression.

Theme

Persecutory delusions are the most frequently encountered and may occur in delirium and schizophrenia, but less often in affective disorders.

- 'Do you believe anyone is trying to harm you?'

Grandiose delusions relate to ideas of exaggerated self-importance and abilities. They are particularly associated with mania.

- 'Do you feel that you have any extraordinary abilities?'
- 'Do you think anyone could have reason to be envious of you?'

Delusions of reference are beliefs that aspects of the environment, e.g. objects, events, people, or communications have a particular significance to the patient. They are suggestive of schizophrenia. The appropriateness of this belief should be explored in order to distinguish from the self-consciousness which some have in social situations. Non-delusional thoughts of this type are termed 'ideas of reference'.

- 'Do you have the feeling that people are talking about you?'
- 'Do you think people mention you on radio, television or in the newspaper?'

Delusions of thought possession: a number of delusional experiences are recognized in which the patient may lose the conviction that their thoughts are private experiences under their own control. They are highly suggestive of schizophrenia and include:

- Thought insertion – the patient believes that some of his/her thoughts have been put into his/her mind from outside.
- Thought withdrawal – the patient believes that some of his/her thoughts have been removed from his/her mind; this may be evident objectively by sudden cessation in the flow of speech known as thought blocking (see above).
- Thought broadcasting – this is the belief that thoughts, though unspoken, may become known to other people by various means, such as thoughts being heard directly by other people; it must be distinguished from the common feeling that others can infer thoughts from a person's actions. 'Do you have difficulty thinking clearly? … Have you had the feeling that perhaps your thoughts were not your own?'

Delusion of control is the belief that actions, impulses, or sensations (somatic passivity) are being controlled and caused by an outside agent. It can be distinguished from command hallucinations which the individual obeys. Delusions of control are sometimes referred to as passivity experiences, and are highly suggestive of schizophrenia. 'Do you ever feel that you are not completely in control of … some of your actions … thoughts … feelings … the functioning of your body?'

Delusions of guilt and worthlessness are associated with severe depressive illness.

- 'Do you feel you are to blame for anything?'

Nihilistic delusions are abnormal beliefs that the patient has ceased to exist, or that something inside has died. It is an unusual delusion, but can be seen in a depressive psychosis.

Delusion of jealousy is the conviction of an individual (usually male) about their partner's infidelity. Their presence is a matter for great concern, as dangerously aggressive behaviour can ensue. Morbid jealousy should be distinguished from less intense and less persistent preoccupations, which are relatively common.

Other delusional themes include **religious, hypochondriacal, and sexual/amorous.**

Perception

- *Déjà vu* phenomena are feelings of having seen or done something before, when in fact the experience is novel. They are associated with complex partial seizures, though they occur in other disorders and can occur as a normal experience.
- Depersonalization and derealization are unpleasant feelings of an altered unreal sense of self or the external world. Although they can occur in the absence of psychiatric illness, they are particularly associated with anxiety disorders.
- Illusions are abnormal perceptions of external stimuli. Visual illusions are associated with delirium and more likely when sensory stimulation is reduced, e.g. poorly lit ward.

Hallucinations These are perceptions in the absence of an external stimulus. They have a similar quality to that of a true perception, i.e. they are perceived in objective space rather than inside the head. Their presence can be suggested by a patient's behaviour, e.g. auditory hallucinations by a patient speaking to themselves. They can occur in any of the five senses. Brief hallucinations when falling asleep (hypnagogic) or while wakening (hypnopompic) are within the range of normal experience. Since some patients may conceal or are unable to express their hallucinations, enquiries should be tactful and sensitive.

Auditory hallucinations are most common and occur in all psychoses, although certain types are particularly associated with schizophrenia.

- 'Have you been having any strange or unusual experiences?'
- 'Do you sometimes hear noises or whispering that no-one else seems to hear?'
- 'Do you sometimes hear someone is speaking to or about you when there is no one else around?'
  Hallucinations can be considered in terms of their:
- Modality (auditory, visual, tactile, olfactory, gustatory).
- Nature (simple or complex).
- Content.

Cognitive assessment (See Chapter 6)

All patients should undergo cognitive screening, although this will vary in complexity depending on the presenting difficulties. If the patient can give a clear and accurate history, there is unlikely to be a cognitive impairment. The aim is to carry out a global assessment of intellectual functioning. Some patients may find the questions very easy, and it is useful to acknowledge this and explain the reason for them, in order to avoid any possible offence being taken. 'I'd like to ask some questions to test your memory and thinking, which are part of the routine assessment; you may find them easy.'

Orientation Is the patient fully alert or is there an impairment of attention, suggesting an acute organic mental disorder (delirium)?

Attention and concentration Digit span: (a test of registration or immediate memory). Ask the patient to repeat a sequence of digits given slowly, both forwards and backwards. The average person should manage six numbers forwards, and five backwards.

Memory
- **Short-term memory:** ask the patient to recall a name and address, learned accurately 5 minutes earlier. Make sure the patient can say it fully and accurately without prompting initially, otherwise the problem could be of registration rather than retention of new material.
- **Long-term memory:** test for current affairs, well-known information, e.g. leaders of state.

Intelligence Simple arithmetic, meanings of words, reading (ask the patient to read the newspaper if there is one to hand).

Tests of specific cortical areas An example is of visuo-spatial awareness. Ask the patient to draw a clock, copy a three-dimensional object, put on an article of clothing (parietal lobe), name objects, or perform abstract reasoning (frontal lobe).

Insight This is the patient's understanding of the nature of his/her problems. The degree of insight varies between patients, and may change over time. Severely restricted insight is a poor prognostic sign which may lead to non-compliance with treatment, and continuation or recurrence of the illness. Attempts to improve insight are an important part of management.

Insight can be assessed using a series of enquiries, the responses to which should be summarized.
- 'What do you think is wrong with you?'
- 'Is the cause within you or something outside?'
- 'Do you think you are ill?'
- 'What do think will help you?'
- 'Do you understand what this treatment is for?'

Physical examination

When psychiatric admission is considered necessary, the responsibility for medical care is transferred to the psychiatric team, and a physical examination and relevant investigations are carried out. However, the possibility of an underlying physical cause should be considered in all psychiatric presentations, and physical examination and investigations performed as indicated.

Key laboratory tests and investigations

Specific tests will be determined by the particular presentation. Commonly ordered investigations are listed in Table 37.

Table 37. Key laboratory tests/investigations

- Thyroid function tests
- Urea and electrolytes (calcium concentration)
- Liver function tests
- Full blood count, plasma viscosity
- Veneral disease reference laboratory (VDRL)
- Hepatitis viral antibodies, HIV counselling and testing
- Therapeutic drug monitoring (lithium, anticonvulsant levels)
- Urine screen for illicit drugs
- EEG
- CT, MRI scans for neuropsychiatric presentations

The following illustrations depict the key features found in anxiety (251), schizophrenia (252), depression (253), and mania (254).

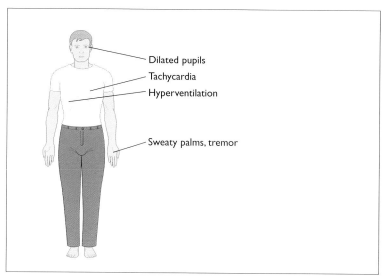

251 Anxiety.

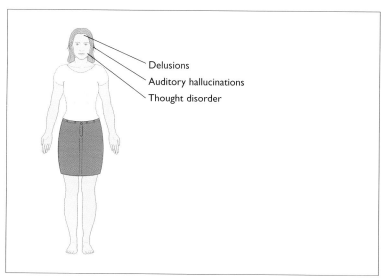

252 Schizophrenia.

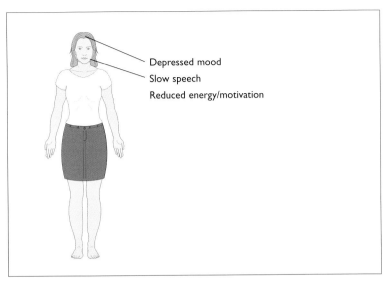

253 Depression.

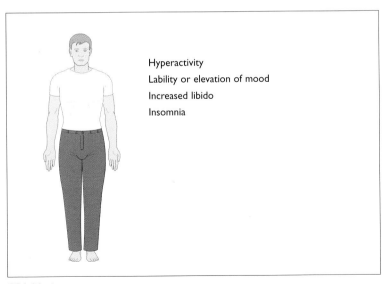

254 Mania.

12 Paediatric history and examination

There is no doubt that the successful examination of a child is more an art than a science, but in order to develop the skills, the same basic knowledge as applies to adults needs to be thoroughly learned. Children get bored quickly and are unable to describe symptoms accurately (if at all). Therefore, one must seize the opportunities as they arise, and not expect an orderly approach. Nevertheless, you need to have an orderly scheme in your mind so as not to miss any signs. The whole process of history-taking and examination need not be stressful if you follow some of the tips given in this chapter.

Legally, a person is classified a 'child' up until the age of 14 years, whence he/she becomes a 'young person' until the age of 17. At 18, they are considered as an adult.

A scheme for history taking and examination of the child

Many of the following tips are common sense to parents, but most medical students and trainee doctors are not parents! Paediatric history taking and examination is time consuming. However, time can be minimized if you spend a few cursory minutes gaining the confidence of the child's parents, and the child's confidence in you. A relaxed, friendly introduction is important, clearly stating your name, position, and your aims. Get everyone seated, or at least comfortable. You need quickly to establish the child's given name, and that by which he/she likes to be called, age, and sex. The latter is not always obvious, and it is better to avoid embarrassment later on. Never refer to a baby as 'it'. Next, determine the relationship of those in the room to the child. It is all too easy to assume big-sister is the mother or – worse still – that the grand-mother is the mother and the real mother the child's sister! Once you have engaged the parents, introduce yourself to the child – preferably using your first-name and his/hers. If the child is very young and

Table 38. Definitions

Description	Age range
Neonate	Birth to 4 weeks (28 days)
Infant	Birth to 1 year
Pre-school	2 to 4+ years
School	5 to 15 years
Childhood period	1 to 15 years
Adolescent period	13 to 19 years

Table 39. History taking and examination in children

The history	The examination
• The presenting complaint	• General observation
• The previous medical history including drug history	• Physical measurements
• The family history	• Examination by systems:
• The social history	– Cardiovascular
• The developmental history	– Chest
	– Abdomen
	– Nervous system

unable to contribute much to the interview, aim to distract him/her with handily placed toys. If the child is older, then you should include him/her in the initial history taking, with frequent affirmations of the parents' details. Watch how the child plays with toys, in particular how the hands and feet are used, eyes and ears, and the way he/she moves. Assess the child's level of anxiety: for example, is he/she happy to leave the mother to play, or does he/she remain in her lap? Is he/she disinterested altogether? If so he/she may be feeling quite ill. All of this visual information will also give you an indication of how best to examine the child later. Try to gauge the gravity of the problem and the parents' concerns early on so that you may behave appropriately. There is little point in bouncing into the consulting room and cracking jokes if a child has been admitted with a first-time grand-mal seizure for example.

Taking the history

Overall, the information sought in a child's medical history is the same as that for an adult, but with a few important additions. You have already ascertained the name, age, and sex of the child – now you need the date of birth, name of the school or nursery he/she attends, where he/she lives (including address and telephone number), and who lives with him/her. You may want to begin with these administrative details, or leave them to the social history section; either way, try to develop your own system so as not to forget to ask for these details. When you first begin history taking you will feel the need to write at the same time as listening, speaking, and looking. This is quite difficult. It's worth asking the patient's/parents' permission, and stopping the interview to do this. Try not to let this interfere with the natural flow of the interview – if needs be, take no notes at this time. Often, experienced paediatricians will write up their notes when the consultation is over.

The presenting complaint

Start by noting the child's or parents' main complaint(s), allowing them to recount in their own way. Only then ask specific questions to clarify important points. It is often a very useful exercise to repeat back to the child or parents these points, to show your understanding of the situation. Try to ascertain the time interval and chronology of events. It is useful to ask when was the last time the child was completely well. If the problem(s) have been going on for some time, determine how much school has been missed, and whether sports and leisure activities have been affected. It is important to enquire about altered patterns of sleep, appetite, and activity as these are often associated with serious illness in children. Ask about weight loss. Is the cry different from normal? With babies, ask what volume of milk is usually taken and actually taken. Try and get a picture of what the child is like when not ill. Is he/she an active child? Does he/she have many friends?

Rather than use a rigid system-by-system barrage of questions, try to concentrate on presenting problems and ask about associated features:

- **Abdominal pain** is a common complaint in babies and children. Babies tend to draw up their legs with abdominal pain, but it must be remembered that this may emanate from anywhere. Toddlers often say that they have 'tummy ache' when asked to localize pain. Enquire about the type of pain and its timing. What aggravates and what relieves it? Is it constant or intermittent? Where does it radiate? Children with chest infections or pneumonia can present with abdominal pain. 'Is there any diarrhoea, constipation, blood in the stools, vomiting, or swelling?'

- **Abdominal distension.** Is it present or absent? Has it been present and resolved?

- **Vomiting.** You need to determine the frequency of vomiting and the volumes each time. The consistency and colour (bile-stained, clear, or bloody) of the vomitus is important. Is it forceful or projectile – possibly indicative of upper gastrointestinal obstruction (i.e. pyloric stenosis). Is it associated with screaming (intussusception), diarrhoea, or pyrexia? In babies, it is important to distinguish normal posseting from true vomiting.

- **Bowel movements.** Ask about the frequency of bowel opening and consistency of the stools, bearing in mind that babies often have semi-solid, mustard-coloured motions. Determine whether there is any accompanying mucus or blood. If there is blood, is it streaky or uniform? Is it dark (malaena) or fresh? What colour are the stools (pale or dark)? Are they difficult to flush away? Is there an unusual odour? Is there pain on defaecation? Does the child soil (encopresis)?

- **Sore throat.** Infants and toddlers are unable to localize pain well, and rarely complain of sore throats.
- **Swallowing** may be painful and lead to refusal to eat. An obstructive or neuromuscular cause usually permits the child to swallow, but shortly after the food is regurgitated.
- **Thirst.** Enquire about the frequency and intensity of thirst (polydipsia is frequent drinking). Is it accompanied by excess urine output (diabetes or renal disease)? What kind of volumes are involved?
- **Micturition.** Is there frequency or urgency? Is this nocturnal or only during the day? Is there accompanying pain (crying or screaming)? What is the colour of the urine (red, dark, clear)? Is there an unusual odour?
- **Bed-wetting** or **day wetting** (enuresis). This is common in young children, and more so in boys up to the age of 10 years. Is there associated polydipsia? If this is a new symptom, have there been any recent events in the child's life which may be connected? Is the child chastised for bed-wetting?
- **Cough** is common. You need to determine its character; is it moist or dry, worse at night, paroxysmal or continuous? Is it associated with chest pain, an inspiratory 'whoop', or wheezing. Is the quality 'barking' (croup)? Is the sputum clear, mucopurulent, or blood-stained?
- **Difficulty in breathing.** Is breathing noisy (wheeze or stridor)? Is it associated with exercise or present at rest? Any exacerbating factors? Is there an associated cough or cyanosis? Does the patient snore or sleep with the mouth open or shut?
- **Cyanosis.** Is this central or confined to the peripheries? Is it intermittent or persistent?
- **Pallor.** Babies are often pale, and even when there is only mild illness can become mottled.
- **Breath.** Does the breath smell of acetone (pear-drops) or is there fetor?
- **Swelling.** Determine the exact size and position, and whether it is increasing or decreasing. Is it painful at rest or just to touch? Is it fluctuant? Is there any associated lymphadenopathy?
- **Rashes/skin lesions.** Ascertain the sight and distribution. Where did it begin? How has it spread? Ask the parents to describe the rash in terms of it colour and morphology – blistering (vesicular), ulcerative, papular (raised), macular (flat), or itchy (pruritic).
- **Jaundice.** How long has this been noted? Has there been any change in the colour of the urine or stools?
- **Musculature.** Enquire as to whether the parents have noted any abnormal movements, or lack of movement. Was the infant floppy at birth? Does the mother find it difficult to handle her child for fear of the child slipping

through her fingers (hypotonia)? On the other hand, is the child stiff (hypertonic/spasticity)? Are there any involuntary movements?

- **Posture.** Is there anything unusual about the child's posture?
- **Coordination.** Is the child unduly clumsy when age is taken into account? Has this always been the case or is this a new phenomenon?
- **Fits** are common in young children and need to be investigated thoroughly. Ask the parents or witness what they saw and describe the type of movements (if any) involved. 'Was there generalized shaking or localized twitching? If so, which limb?' 'Was the child unconscious? Did he/she vomit or bite their tongue? How long did the episode last? How long was the child unconscious for after the fits ceased? Has this ever happened before? Did the child hit his head before the fit, or as a consequence of it? Was the child incontinent? Was there any indication of a preceding aura or pyrexia?'
- **Speech.** Was there any delay in onset of speech? Is there any residual language or speech articulation problem? Once speech was achieved, was there any subsequent loss of speech? Ask whether the child has ever had speech therapy?
- **Vision.** If a baby, have the parents noted whether he/she is able to follow an object held close up? In older children, is there any difficulty in reading or seeing the blackboard at school? Does the child bump into things in subdued light (night blindness)?
- **Hearing.** Are there any concerns about hearing?
- **Behaviour.** Is the child active or hyperactive, or is he/she quiet or apathetic? How would the parents describe the child: aggressive or placid, gregarious or a loner, obedient or disobedient? If a toddler, does he/she have frequent temper tantrums, nightmares, sleep-walking, or night-time waking? How does the rest of the household cope with these problems, and what has been done to improve them so far?

In this section, ask the parents what they think is causing the problem(s). They may save you a lot of unnecessary questions, examining, and investigations.

Past medical history

Try to collect information in some kind of order. A chronological order of events is the easiest to remember.

Pregnancy and birth Begin at the beginning with the mother's pregnancy (single or multiple) and labour. Were there any maternal infections or illnesses? Was the baby born at term (40 weeks) or preterm (usually written 30/40, if born at 30 weeks)? Was the delivery vaginal or caesarean? If the latter was it elective (why) or emergency (why)? Was the presentation normal vertex or breech, or

Table 40. The APGAR score

Sign	Score		
	1	2	3
Colour	Blue/pale	Pink trunk, blue extremities	Pink all over
Heart rate	Absent	<100	>100
Reflex irritability	None	Grimace	Cry
Tone	Limp	Some limb flexion	Active movement
Respiratory effort	Absent	Slow, irregular	Strong cry

assisted by forceps or Ventouse (suction) extraction? What was the baby's condition at birth (if the mother has the child's community record book to hand, check the APGAR scores)? What was the birth weight? How were the first few days of life (jaundiced or special care)? Was he/she breast or bottle-fed and when was he/she weaned? Were there any feeding problems?

APGAR scoring This is a validated scoring system for assessing the health of a neonate. The total score (maximum 10) is usually assessed at 1 and 5 minutes after birth. A low score of <5 at 5 minutes is associated with long-term developmental problems (see **Table 40**).

Drug history and allergies Has the child received any medication for the current problems? Is he/she on any long-term drugs? State the generic name, as well as the trade name, in all cases. Record the dose and frequency of administration, not just what was prescribed.

Does the child have any allergies to drugs, house-dust mite, cats, dogs, fur, nuts, shellfish? What happens when he/she is exposed to the antigen? Is there any history of acute anaphylaxis or rash?

Infections or illnesses Which common childhood infections/exanthemas has the child had? Any hospital admissions? Where, date, and duration? Any recent contact with infectious persons or animals (including birds)?

Recent travel or residence abroad Obtain details of which countries, and whether resident in town or rural location (malaria for example is seldom found in large towns).

Immunizations An immunization history must be sought, noting whether it is up-to-date. The triple vaccine (DPT) is often called the '3-in-1'. Ask about polio vaccine (Sabin vaccine on a sugar-lump or drop on the tongue). Don't forget to ask about BCG and hepatitis B and C, no matter what the age or race of the child, as well as mumps, measles and rubella (MMR) and *Haemophilus influenzae* (Hib) vaccine. You must know the standard vaccination regimen. Has the child had any inoculations related to foreign travel (cholera, typhoid)?

Family history

Determine the relationship of all members of the immediate family. The construction of a family tree will help in organizing your questions and records. In this you should record the age and state of health of each sibling and parent. Is the parents' union consanguineous? If so to what degree? Have there been any childhood deaths or stillbirths? Are there any hereditary disorders in the family? Ask about thalassaemia and sickle cell disease if the patient is not Caucasian.

Social history

This is a sensitive part of the interview, and there is no way easy way of asking the relevant questions. Most people do not mind answering these if you explain their importance. You need to know who works in the family? What are the members' occupations? Are there any hazards? Who smokes cigarettes/pipe/cigars? What is the overall mood in the household? Are there any conflicts, separations, or divorces? Who else lives in the house other than immediate family (note their name and sex in cases of suspected abuse)? Try and ascertain the size and condition of the home. Is there heating, running water, and adequate sanitation? Try and determine how well the child is doing at school. Is he/she reluctant to go to school in the mornings? Is the child being bullied? The child may be happy to tell you, a stranger, about these problems which they might not mention to their own family.

Developmental history

Developmental milestones are divided into four broad categories:
1 Social.
2 Hearing and speech.
3 Vision and fine motor skills.
4 Gross motor skills.

Try to learn at least two features from each category at key ages (i.e. 6 weeks, 6 months, 1 year, 18 months, 2 years, 3 years, 4 years and 5 years).

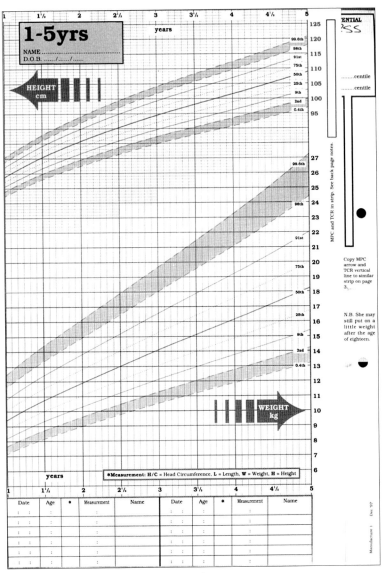

255 Growth chart for weight of girls aged 1–5.

The examination

How you approach the examination depends on the age of the child. The eldest will be no different from the adult. However, younger children are not so straightforward. Approach the child with a quiet voice and warm hands. Next – and this is most important – get down to the child's level, even if this means on your hands and knees. The examination is just as daunting for the child as for you. Keep your examination equipment out of sight, or you will rapidly lose a friend before you have even begun. Introduce the stethoscope, and allow the patient to play with it. Babies of 1–3 months are surprisingly cooperative if you remember to smile and speak quietly. Probably the easiest age for examination is between 6 and 10 months, when all babies are friendly. Unfortunately, by about 10 months they have learned to be suspicious of strangers, and remain so throughout their time as a toddler. This age group is the most difficult, and they need to be distracted by making a game of the examination. Let them play with your stethoscope or pen-torch. Toddlers don't like to be stared at, and will usually avoid direct eye contact. From 5 years onwards, children become more cooperative again, and are less reluctant to leave their parents' side. Always talk to the child, and not at him/her. Try to break the ice by talking about something topical in the child's life, such as a favourite toy, pop group, or TV programme. If the patient is very young, ask the parents to help undress the child down to the underwear at first. The rest can come off in stages. Begin by touching the child's hands, and even play a game such as 'this little piggy' to win his/her confidence. Demonstrate auscultation, auroscopy, or ophthalmoscopy on an adult or doll first. Leave the examination of the ears, nose, throat, and rectum until the end. Babies dislike having their head circumference measured, and it may be wise to leave this until later.

Physical measurements

Do these first, so as not to forget them.

- **Height/length:** obtain measurements of crown–rump length, as this is easier to perform and more reliable than crown–heel. Use a measuring board if available. Children who can stand need to be measured against a wall-mounted rule, with their shoes removed. Plot values on age- and sex-related charts and note the nearest percentile. If you are worried about limb length or asymmetry measure both limbs for comparison. For upper limbs, measure from the tip of the acromion process to the tip of the middle finger. For lower limbs, measure from the anterior superior iliac spine to the internal malleolus.
- **Weight (255):** a new-born baby will normally lose 10–15% of the birth weight within the first week of life. They should have regained their birth

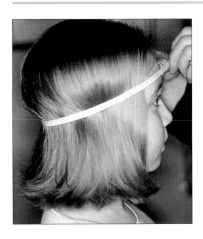

256 Measuring the head circumference of a girl.

weight by 10 days. The average weight gain in the first 3 months is about 25 g (~1 oz) per day. Infants usually double their birth weight by 5 months, and treble it by one year. A quick formula for estimating the weight of a child between 1 and 9 years of age is:

Weight (kg) = (Age [in years] + 4) × 2

Again, these values need to be plotted on standard charts and the nearest percentile noted.

Head circumference (OFC) Measurements are made at the level of the supra-orbital ridges and the occipital protuberance (**256**). Plot these on standard charts.

Blood pressure Auscultatory blood pressure measurements may be taken using a cuff and sphygmomanometer in 3-year-olds and older. Child-sized cuffs are readily available (usually 5 cm and 7.5 cm), and when applied should cover two-thirds of the upper arm. In younger children and babies the palpatory methods can be employed. In difficult cases such as dehydration and hypovolaemia, Doppler ultrasound blood pressure monitors are now available. Normal blood pressure values are:

- New-born   75/50 mmHg
- Infants   80/55 mmHg (± 20%)
- Pre-school   85/60 mmHg
- School child   90/60 mmHg

Temperature In babies, a thermometer may be placed in the groin crease, axilla, or rectum. In older children, the axilla is preferred (children cannot resist biting

Examining the cardiovascular system

Approximately 1% of new-born babies will have a congenital heart defect. However, only about half of these will be detectable at birth.

● **Inspection.** Start with the peripheries and work your way centrally towards the heart. Note cyanosis, clubbing, tachypnoea, pallor (anaemia), or polycythaemia. Watch for a visible precordial heave or lift due to heart enlargement (left ventricular hypertrophy (LVH) – apical region; right ventricular hypertrophy (RVH) – sternal/parasternal). The jugular venous pressure (JVP) is very difficult to determine in young children due to the shortness of the neck.

● **Pulses.** Feel for the radial, brachial, and femoral arteries bilaterally, using your finger-tips and pressing lightly at first. It is easy to miss a pulse through total occlusion. The femoral pulses are often difficult to find, but do persist as a truly absent pulse may be indicative of coarctation of the aorta. Go on to look for radiofemoral delay. If you can feel a dorsalis-pedis in an infant, they do not have coarctation. Don't forget to place a hand over the scapulae if you suspect a coarctation – you may feel the pulsation of collateral vessels.

  Determine whether the pulse volume is normal, large, or small. Sinus arrhythmia is accentuated, but normal in children (increased heart rate on inspiration and decrease on expiration). A large 'bounding' pulse may indicate a hyperdynamic circulation associated with shunting. A feeble, low-volume pulse may indicate left outflow tract restriction. A collapsing 'water-hammer' pulse is associated with aortic regurgitation.

---

a glass thermometer). If hypothermia is suspected, a low-reading thermometer (29–43°C) should be placed in the rectum. Recently infrared devices have been developed in which an unobtrusive ear probe is placed in the external auditory meatus for 1 second, and the reflected heat of the tympanic membrane is measured directly. Normal temperature values are:

● Normal infant skin   37°C
● Normal infant rectum   38°C
● Premature baby   36°C

Examination by systems
Here, a detailed description is provided of the examination of an infant and older child. For details of the neonatal examination, the reader should refer to a textbook of neonatology. The general order for examination is as follows: inspection, percussion, palpation, auscultation.

Precordium

The apex beat is best felt with the pulp tip of the third finger of the right hand lightly resting on the left 4th or 5th intercostal space between the mid-clavicular and mid-axillary lines (**257**).

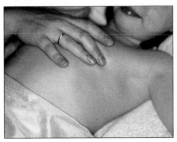

257 Listening for the apex beat.

Praecordial pulsations of LVH and RVH and cardiac thrills are best appreciated with the palm of the hand.

● **Percussion.** Unlike the adult, percussion of the cardiac borders can be easily achieved in children due to the thinness of the thoracic cage. The right cardiac border should not extend beyond the right border of the sternum. The upper cardiac border should not be felt above the 2nd intercostal space.

● **Auscultation.** It is acceptable to use the bell throughout auscultatory examination of young children. However, in difficult situations the second heart sound is often best heard with the diaphragm over the pulmonary area. A systematic examination should begin by listening over the mitral area (apex), the pulmonary area (2nd left costal cartilage), the aortic area (in the 1st and 2nd intercostal spaces at the right sternal edge), and the tricuspid area (along the left lower sternal edge at about the 4th intercostal space). Listen for radiation of murmurs; mitral systolic into the left axilla; aortic systolic into the neck; aortic systolic down the left sternal edge. Physiological splitting of the second heart sound is commonly heard at the pulmonary area on inspiration in children and young adults. A third heart sound is also commonly heard, especially at the apex, and is entirely normal in the young. This should be differentiated from a pathological second sound splitting which is more widely spaced (and quieter) than the physiological split. Other sounds to note are the presence of a gallop rhythm (heart failure) and a pericardial rub.

Examining the respiratory system

Look at the shape of the chest. Note the presence of any deformities such as pectus excavatum, pectus carinatum (pigeon-chest), Harrison's sulci (chronic severe asthma), costochondral junction swelling (rickety-rosary), or dinner-fork deformity (scurvy).

Measure the respiratory rate at rest:
- 0–2 years   40 per minute
- 2–6 years   30 per minute
- 6–10 years   25 per minute
- >10 years   20 per minute

Inspiratory time is normally longer than the expiratory phase, but in children they are often equal. Is there prolonged expiration as in asthma? Is there any intercostal indrawing or costal recession indicative of airflow obstruction? Are there any upper airways noises such as stridor (inspiratory or expiratory), grunting (infants), or wheezing?

- **Percussion.** Chest percussion in the child is more resonant than in the adult, and it is relatively easy to determine dullness.

- **Auscultation.** Due to the equality of the inspiratory and expiratory phases, breath sounds in children are bronchovesicular. Breath sounds may be decreased in bronchiolitis, pneumothorax, severe asthma, pleural effusion, collapse, or emphysema. They may be increased in consolidation of the lung. The wheeze of asthma tends to be high-pitched and 'musical'. Listen for a pleural rub.

    Vocal resonance may be diminished in pleural effusion and increased in consolidation. Whispering pectoriloquy may be heard with consolidation.

Examining the abdomen

Begin with the hands, looking for signs of anaemia, clubbing, leukonychia, and spider naevi. Note any distention of the abdomen, and whether there is accompanying venous congestion indicative of liver disease (and ascites). Look for visible peristalsis which may be associated with obstruction. Are the hernial orifices swollen (including the umbilicus – **258** and **259**)?

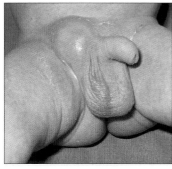

258 Inguinal hernia.

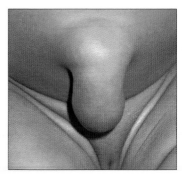

259 Umbilical hernia.

● **Palpation.** Place the patient flat on the couch or in the parent's arms. Kneel down so as to be on a level with the child's abdomen, and warm your hands. Begin by using your right hand with light palpation in all four quadrants to determine whether there are any areas of tenderness. Often if you ask a young child (e.g. toddler) whether he/she has pain, he/she will invariably answer in the affirmative – which may be unhelpful. Always watch the patient's face. If there is tenderness, test for rebound by sudden withdrawal of the hand on deep palpation. If pain is severe, there may be abdominal guarding or even board-like rigidity. If there is mild or no tenderness, proceed with deeper palpation of specific organs. We suggest you begin with the spleen. In young children, the spleen enlarges into the left iliac fossa, whereas in older children and young adults it tends to enlarge across the mid-line to the right iliac fossa. Work your way up into the left hypochondrium until you can just tip the spleen on inspiration. Concomitant placement of your left hand in the child's left renal angle and lifting gently will facilitate identification of the spleen.

Examining the abdomen – continued

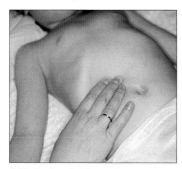

260 Feeling the liver edge.

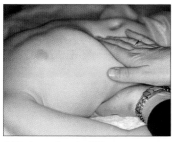

261 Assessing the kidneys.

Next, identify the sharp hepatic edge on inspiration beginning in the right iliac fossa and working upwards toward the right costal margin. The liver edge is normally felt one finger-breadth below the costal margin in young children (**260**).

The kidneys are best balloted between the two hands, with the left placed behind the child in the renal angle and the right hand on the right hypochondrium (**261**).

Palpate the suprapubic region for a distended bladder. A pyloric mass will be felt in the right hypochondrium close to the mid-line, and is best elicited with the child bottle-feeding. An intussusception is sausage-shaped and felt in the right upper quadrant during abdominal relaxation. If ascites are suspected, try and elicit a fluid thrill.

• **Percussion.** This may be helpful in determining the borders of the liver. If there is a suspicion of free fluid in the abdomen, percuss for dullness in the flank, with the patient supine. If present, turn the child onto the left side and percuss again to determine whether there is shifting dullness.

• **Auscultation.** Bowel sounds may be loud following a feed (borborygmi), or tinkling in partial obstruction. They are usually absent in complete obstruction or ileus.

Examination of the nervous system

A formal systematic examination of the nervous system is extremely difficult in the very young child, and this is due in part to lack of cooperation but mainly to immaturity of the system itself. Observation – particularly during certain activities – is the most useful form of examination, and forms the basis of the developmental assessment. Examination is not very different from the adult, and we present some useful reminders under relevant headings.

● **Inspection.** Assess the level of consciousness of the child, and whether he/she is irritable or drowsy.

Next, note the posture at rest and during movement. Are there any abnormal spontaneous movements such as writhing (choreoathetosis) of the upper limbs? Is purposeful, voluntary movement normal? Is there any tremor or clumsiness?

Look at the posture while the child is sitting and standing. Are there any abnormalities of gait? Describe them; broad-based walk of ataxia; stiff scissor-like movements of spasticity; high-stepping gait associated with foot-drop.

If the child is speaking, try to assess the level of speech. Is it appropriate for the child's age? Is articulation of speech normal? Is there monotony or stammering? Try and determine the child's use of language, as this gives an indication of intelligence.

● **Cranial nerves.** These will only be partially examinable in the young. In older children the same adult format should be followed.
Power: the same grading for power is used as for adult medicine (see Chapter 6).
Sensation: the dermatomal distribution in children is the same as that in adults (Chapter 6).

● **Reflexes.** Primitive reflexes may be categorized by age as follows:
2 months – palmar grasp lost; stepping reflex lost.
6 months – Moro reflex lost; asymmetric tonic neck reflex lost.
12 months – Babinski response becomes flexor (down-going).
5 years – Galant response lost (stimulation along a paravertebral line leads to lateral spinal flexion toward the stimulated side).

Other reflexes have the same root innervations as adults (Chapter 6).

Examination of the genitalia

In females, look for labial symmetry, clitoral enlargement, abnormalities of the introitus, and position of the urethra. Note any bruising to the inner thighs, labia, and introitus (see below, Non-accidental injury).
In males, note the size of the penis, the position of the urethra (hypospadias), and the condition of the prepuce (phimosis or balanitis). Examine for the presence of testes in the scrotum. If not palpable, determine their position in the inguinal tract, noting whether or not they are retractable.

Rectal examination

This should be reserved until last. Inspect the anus for correct position, atresia, stenosis, or fissure. Place a gloved and well-lubricated finger (appropriate to the size of the child) into the rectum and sweep around in a clockwise direction, noting areas of tenderness (as in appendicitis) and the presence of pelvic or adnexal masses. Note the presence of any blood on withdrawal.

Child abuse

Classification of child abuse is as follows:

- Non-accidental injury (NAI).
- Neglect and emotional deprivation.
- Failure-to-thrive.
- Sexual abuse.
- Poisoning.
- Munchausen syndrome by proxy.

Non-accidental injury (NAI) This is the most common form of abuse in children and appears to be on the increase (262). Paediatricians are often called upon by the police, social services, GPs, and teachers

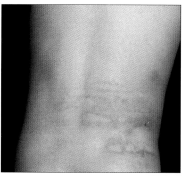

262 Non-accidental injury. Beware of unexplained or poorly explained scars.

to examine a child whom they suspect may be a victim of abuse. As a junior doctor, you should be aware of some of the tell-tale signs of NAI (see box opposite).

Is the child unkempt and unwashed? Is the clothing in a reasonable state and appropriate for the current climate? Has the nappy been changed recently, or is there severe nappy area rash? Is the hair uncombed or are there head-lice?

If sexual abuse is suspected on general examination, do not continue with a genital or rectal examination. Inform the social services and the senior paediatrician, and leave the final examination to the police surgeon or designated gynaecologist.

Note that trauma to the perineum is common in children due to straddling injuries, and the child will usually give detailed account of their misadventure.

Munchausen syndrome by proxy This is the term given to an indirect form of abuse where a parent may report a fictitious illness, injury, or fits in an attempt to get a child treated in hospital in some way (even operated on). The reasons for such behaviour are complex, and beyond the scope of this description. If a child appears to have been seen by several hospitals or specialists with many different ailments, consider this to be a possibility.

Therapeutic and interventional skills
Practical procedures in children and babies
Venepuncture Practical procedures in children can be stressful for the child and doctor alike. This need not be so if a few basic tenets are adhered to. Always ask a nurse or colleague to help you.

- Explain calmly and confidently to the parents and child that you need to perform a procedure (you need not go into details just yet). Do this before approaching the bedside armed with needle and syringe. Explain that it will hurt a little, but for a short period only.
- In the case of small children it may be beneficial to apply a local anaesthetic cream (EMLA or Ametop) to the sample site(s), bearing in mind that these often take up to 1 h to have an effect.
- If there is a designated area for procedures, try to avoid performing them at the child's bedside. After all, this is their temporary home.

Toddlers and babies will need to be restrained. This can be done by sitting the child on the nurse's or mother's lap, with the non-sampling arm firmly pressed against the adult's chest. The arm (or leg) to be sampled then needs to be firmly (but not tightly) held by a second helper, who can also apply mild tourniquet pressure to bring forth the veins. Occasionally, it is useful to use a sheet to wrap around the child in such a way as to immobilize the arms and legs.

History of non-accidental injury

• Bony fractures are unusual in infants under 18 months of age. The exceptions are birth injuries (usually humerus or clavicle evident on X-ray) and brittle bone disease (osteogenesis imperfecta – look for blue sclera).

• Try and ascertain whether the explanation is consistent with severity and site of injury. If a fracture is ascribed to a fall, ask about distance the child fell. Falling off a bed or sofa (under 1 m [3 ft]) will very rarely result in a fracture (and certainly not multiple ones).

• Have there been several attendances at your hospital, other hospitals, or the GP's surgery in recent years?

• Is there an entry on the child protection register ('At-risk register')?

• If asked to repeat the story, does it change subtly each time it is recounted?

• Has there been a delay in presentation (>48 hours)?

Examination for suspected non-accidental injury

With the help of another doctor or nurse, always fully undress the patient, drawing and measuring any injuries. Plot height and weight (and head circumference in babies).

• Look for an unusual distribution of bruising; to the back of the head, neck, trunk, lower back, and buttocks. Bear in mind that young children will invariably have bruises on the lower legs and knees, and toddlers often knock the forehead.

• Accidental fractures are usually transverse or greenstick, and located distally on the affected limb. Skull fractures are usually simple if caused by a fall. Multiple rib fractures (not associated with cycle/car accident) are a common sign of NAI. Suspicious limb fractures are often spiral due to a twisting or pulling action. A depressed skull fracture may be due to a blunt instrument.

• Determine the relative ages of multiple bruises. Are they consistent with the story given? Likewise, with multiple fractures, determine whether they are of differing ages (callus on X-rays).

• 'Highly suspicious injuries' include a torn frenulum in bottle-fed babies; cigarette burns; black eyes; hand-shaped or finger-shaped markings; bite-marks (size will tell you whether it is an adult bite); bruises to the inner thigh or genitals; scalds, especially on the lower limbs and in babies (placed in hot bath). A subdural haematoma is always suspicious.

Occasionally, veins are reluctant to show themselves, particularly if the child is cold or 'shut down'. You can try to place the limb concerned in a bowl of warm water to encourage venodilatation. Note, however, that blood taken in this way will have been 'arterialized', and may affect the outcome of the laboratory tests.

Sampling can now be started (see box below). Remember, gloves must always be worn.

Capillary sampling

This method is suitable for obtaining small quantities of blood, particularly from new-born babies. The side of the heel is cleaned with 70% ethanol and may be smeared with a very thin layer of petroleum jelly to facilitate a smooth flow. A stylet is used vertically to produce the cut. Gently squeeze the foot to encourage blood flow, and hold the siliconized, heparinized capillary tube at about 30° to the horizontal against the bleb of blood. This will flow easily along the tube. If the tube is held too vertically, unwanted air bubbles may be introduced.

Venepuncture

Suitable superficial veins are found in the antecubital fossa, back of the hand, dorsum of the foot, or the scalp. Clean the skin thoroughly with 70% ethanol or chlorhexidine if cultures are to be taken. The sharpened, bevelled end of a broken needle (**263**, below) is inserted into the vein until the tip

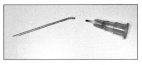

becomes just invisible; blood should then begin to flow as individual droplets, which can be collected directly into bottles. The flow can be encouraged by gentle squeezing of the hand. In difficult situations, the scalp vein may be sampled, in which case a butterfly needle should be used.

In older children, a butterfly needle (23-gauge) should be used, with a 5-ml syringe attached. Before sampling, secure the wings of the butterfly with tape, as invariably the needle will pull out.

On extraction of the needle, always apply firm pressure for at least 1 minute to prevent haematoma formation.

Intravenous cannulation

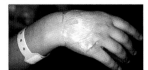

Following local anaesthetic application (264), clean the skin thoroughly with 70% ethanol or chlorhexidine.

264 Application of local anaesthetic.

The following equipment is required (265):

- A cannula (22–24 gauge) with short wings.
- Fixing tape (~1 cm wide).
- Splint and bandage.
- One 2-ml syringe filled with 0.9% saline.
- Extension tubing flushed with saline.

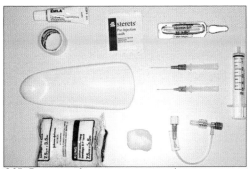

265 Equipment for intravenous cannulation.

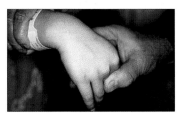

Ideal veins for cannulation include the median cubital vein, or a dorsal hand vein with a Y-junction (266). These veins are relatively immobile.

Continued overleaf

266 Checking veins for cannulation.

Intravenous cannulation – continued

Proceed as follows:

● Get a colleague to apply gentle tourniquet pressure proximal to the vein.

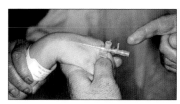

267 Checking for flashback.

● Pierce the skin about 0.5 cm distal to the intended site of entry into the vein. Push the cannula forward in the subcutaneous tissue until you reach the Y-junction (or chosen entry site), and aim to enter the vein from above. You will know when the needle is in the vessel lumen by the flashback in the hub (**267**).

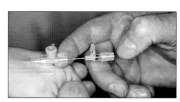

268 Inserting the cannula.

● Now advance the needle very gently a little further, so that the cannula itself is situated in the lumen (**268**). Carefully hold the cannula hub stationary with one hand while withdrawing the needle with the other hand. If the needle is still in the vein, blood will flow back down the hub.

● Gently advance the cannula into the vein until it is no longer visible on the skin surface.

● Insert the primed extension piece into the hub and flush the lumen with 1 ml of saline. Cap off the extension piece.

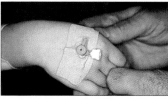

269 Securing the cannula with tape.

● Fix the wings of the cannula securely with two strips of tape (**269**). Apply the splint to the contralateral surface of the limb and tape into place, allowing the entry site to be clearly visible.

● In younger children it may be necessary to bandage the splint to prevent pulling and playing. Now run through a 'giving-set' with the desired fluid and connect it to the extension piece.

Glossary of commonly used abbreviations

↑	Increased
→	Deviated towards the right
↓	Decreased
A2	Aortic component of second heart sound
AB	Apex beat
AC	Air conduction
ACTH	Adrenocorticotrophic hormone
ADH	Antidiuretic hormone
AF	Atrial fibrillation
AFB	Acid-fast bacilli
AJ	Ankle jerk
ALP	Alkaline phosphatase
ALT	Alanine amino transferase
Anti-DNA	Antibody characteristic of SLE
APGAR	Dr Virginia Apgar
AS	Added sounds / Alimentary system / Aortic stenosis / Ankylosing spondylitis
ASD	Atrial septal defect
AST	Aspartate amino transferase
AVF/AVL/AVR	ECG leads looking from right arm (AVR), left arm (AVL), and feet (AVF)
AVP	Arginine vasopressin
BC	Bone conduction
BCG	Bacille Calmette Guerin – the vaccination against tuberculosis
BJ	Biceps jerk
BMI	Body mass index
Bp	Blood pressure
bpm	Beats per minute
BS	Breath sounds / Bowel sounds
BSV	Breath sounds vesicular
C/O	Complains of
CCF	Congestive cardiac failure
CE	Cardiac enzymes
CK	Creatine kinase
CMC	Carpometacarpal joint
CNS	Central nervous system
COAD	Chronic obstructive airways disease
COPD	Chronic obstructive pulmonary disease
CSF	Cerebrospinal fluid
CT	Computed tomography
CVA	Cerebrovascular accident
CVP	Central venous pressure
CVS	Cardiovascular system
CXR	Chest X-ray
D/N	Day/night in relation to frequency of micturition
DPT	Diphtheria, polio, tetanus vaccine (triple vaccine)
DVT	Deep vein thrombosis
ECG	Electrocardiogram

EEG	Electroencephalogram
EMLA	Topical anaesthetic cream
ENA	Extractable nuclear antigens
ESR	Erythrocyte sedimentation rate
FBC	Full blood count
FH	Family history
γGT	Gamma glutamyl transferase
GALS	Gait, arms, legs, spine
GIS / GIT	Gastrointestinal system
GTN	Glyceryl trinitrate
GUS	Genitourinary system
HAP	Heart apex beat
Hb	Haemoglobin
HbeAg	Hepatitis B e antigen
HbsAg	Hepatitis B surface antigen
Hib	*Haemophilus influenzae*
HPC	History of the present condition
HS	Heart sounds
Hx	History
ICS	Intercostal space
Ig	Immunoglobulin
IHD	Ischaemic heart disease
INR	International normalized ratio
IUCD	Intrauterine contraceptive device
i.v.	Intravenous
JVP	Jugular venous pressure
KJ	Knee jerk
kPa	Kilo Pascals
KY®	A commercially available lubricant jelly
LBBB	Left bundle branch block
LCF	Left ventricular failure
LFTs	Liver function tests
LIF	Left iliac fossa
LMP	Last menstrual period
LN	Lymph nodes
LSD	Lysergic acid diethylamide
LSKK	Liver, spleen, and kidneys
LVF	Left ventricular failure
LVH	Left ventricular hypertrophy
MCP	Metacarpophalangeal joint
MI	Myocardial infarction
mmHg	Millimeters of mercury
MMR	Measles, mumps, rubella
MRC	Medical Research Council
MRI	Magnetic resonance imaging
MS	Mitral stenosis / Multiple sclerosis
MSE	Mental state examination
MSS	Musculoskeletal system
MTP	Metatarsophalangeal joint
NAD	No abnormality detected
NAI	Non-accidental injury
NS	Nervous system
NSU	Non-specific urethritis
O/E	On examination
OFC	Head circumference
OS	Opening snap (heart sound)

P	Pulse
P/C	Presenting complaint
P2	Pulmonary component of second heart sound
PaO_2	Partial pressure of oxygen
PA	Postero-anterior / Pulmonary artery
$PaCO_2$	Partial pressure of carbon dioxide
PE	Pulmonary emboli
PEFR	Peak expiratory flow rate
PERLA	Pupils equal, react to light and accommodation
PH	Personal history
PMH	Past medical history
PN	Percussion note
POMR	Problem-oriented medical records
PP	Peripheral pulses
PR	Per rectum / Plantar response
PT	Prothrombin time
PTTK	Partial thromboplastin time
QRS	The wave form of the ECG
Reflexes: B	biceps
T	triceps
S	supinator
K	knee
A	ankle
P	plantar response
RIF	Right iliac fossa
RIH	Right inguinal hernia
ROS	Review of systems
RS	Respiratory system
RVH	Right ventricular hypertrophy
S1	First heart sound
S2	Second heart sound
SBE	Subacute bacterial endocarditis / Standard base excess
SH	Social history
SHO	Senior house officer
SIADH	Syndrome of inappropriate antidiuretic hormone secretion
SLE	Systemic lupus erythematosus
SM	An antibody characteristic of SLE
SOA	Swelling of ankles
SOAPI	Subjective, objective, assessment, plan, and information
SOBE	Short of breath on exertion
SVC	Superior vena cava
SVT	Supraventricular tachycardia
TB	Tuberculosis
TH	Treatment history
TJ	Triceps jerk
TT	Thrombin time
TVF	Tactile vocal fremitus
Tx	Treatment
U&E	Plasma urea and electrolyte concentration
VDRL	Venereal Disease Reference Laboratory
VP	Venous pressure
VR	Vocal resonance
WBC	White blood cell count

Index